World Histories of Crime, Culture and Violence

Palgrave's World Histories of Crime, Culture and Violence seeks to publish research monographs, collections of scholarly essays, multi-authored books, and Palgrave Pivots addressing themes and issues of interdisciplinary histories of crime, criminal justice, criminal policy, culture and violence globally and on a wide chronological scale (from the ancient to the modern period). It focuses on interdisciplinary studies, historically contextualized, across various cultures and spaces employing a wide range of methodologies and conceptual frameworks.

More information about this series at
http://www.springer.com/series/14383

Zahira Aragüete-Toribio

Producing History in Spanish Civil War Exhumations

From the Archive to the Grave

palgrave
macmillan

Zahira Aragüete-Toribio
University of Geneva
Geneva, Switzerland

World Histories of Crime, Culture and Violence
ISBN 978-3-319-61269-0 ISBN 978-3-319-61270-6 (eBook)
DOI 10.1007/978-3-319-61270-6

Library of Congress Control Number: 2017944590

Cover illustration: Game pieces found in mass grave, Puebla de Alcocer, 2012. © Zahira Aragüete Toribio

Printed on acid-free paper

This Palgrave Macmillan imprint is published by Springer Nature
The registered company is Springer International Publishing AG
The registered company address is: Gewerbestrasse 11, 6330 Cham, Switzerland

Map of Extremadura

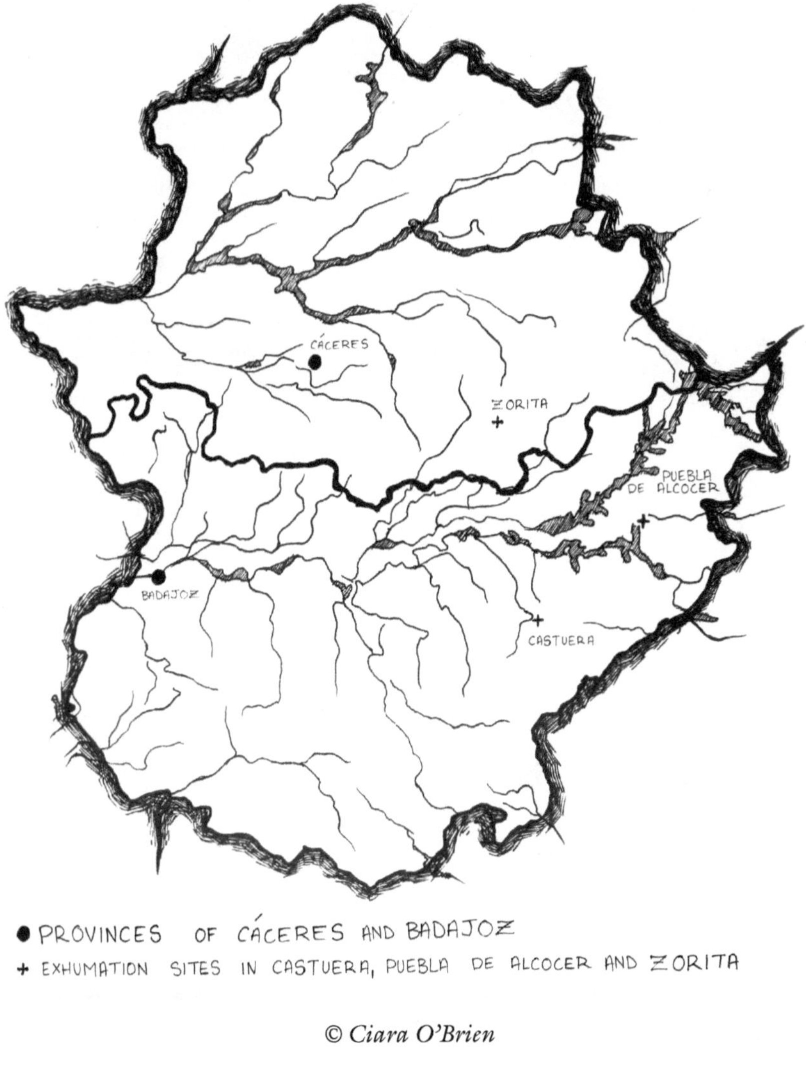

© *Ciara O'Brien*

For Maria and Piedad

Acknowledgements

This book would not have been possible without the ongoing trust and encouragement of many people and the support of different institutions. My field research carried out between December 2010 and September 2012 and my Ph.D. thesis, on which this monograph is based, were part of the project *Bosnian Bones, Spanish Ghosts: Transitional Justice and the Legal Shaping of Memory after Two Modern Conflicts*, funded by the European Research Council and led by Dr. Sari Wastell at Goldsmiths, University of London, United Kingdom. The publication of the manuscript could have not been possible without the support of the project *Right to Truth, Truth(s) through Rights: Mass Crimes Impunity and Transitional Justice*, funded by the Swiss National Science Foundation and led by Professor Sévane Garibian at the University of Geneva, Switzerland. I thank both projects and their teams for allowing me to be part of years of enriching learning and research.

The extensive fieldwork I conducted in Extremadura and my participation in different exhumations was indeed possible thanks to the collaboration of many associations, families and institutional initiatives. I thank the Project for the Recovery of Historical Memory in Extremadura (PREMHEx) and its project director until 2014, Julián Chaves Palacios, for his warm welcome and for allowing me to follow the team's activities. I thank its members at that time, Cayetano Ibarra Barroso, Laura Muñoz Encinar, Candela Chaves Rodriguez, Javier Martin Bastos, and Inés Belén Fernández, for their extreme generosity, for teaching me the craft of the historian and the archaeologist, and for our enlightening conversations. I am eternally grateful to the different teams of volunteers I collaborated with at distinct sites. Their passion, their amity, and their laughter turned every excavation campaign into a unique experience.

In Castuera, the Association for the Memory of Castuera Concentration Camp or AMECADEC kindly invited me to participate in the exhumation they promoted in 2011. I thank its then president Guillermo León Cáceres and historian Antonio López Rodriguez for sharing their extensive knowledge about the Camp and the repression in the area with me. This book is dedicated to the memory of Aurora Navas Morillo and to Maria Hormeño, Marielo Gil, and Ángel Sayabera for opening their homes and sharing their private worlds with me. In Puebla de Alcocer, I thank the group of families that promoted the exhumation carried out in the village in 2012 and the family of José Sánchez-Paniagua for their hospitality and care. My knowledge of the history of the war in the locality would have not been the same without the stories of José, his sister Consuelo and their father José, and also those of Luisa Cabanillas Bayón, Esperanza Muga Blasco, Pablo Trenado Cabanillas, Emiliano Bayón Villarejo, Mariano, and José Gómez Mayoral, Begoña, and Jacinto Velasco. In Garciaz, I thank the association led by Javier Martin Bastos in 2011 and its family members for making me part of their ongoing search for the human remains of their relatives in the village of Zorita. In Badajoz, I am grateful for the constant help of the Association for the Recovery of Historical Memory in Extremadura (ARMHEx) and its president José Manuel Corbacho. I am also grateful to José Hinojosa Durán and AMECECA and to historians José Maria Lama and Francisco Cebrián for generously providing me with an insight into their work and sharing their records with me. I thank Libertad González Barroso for kindly retelling her father's story and her family's biography to me.

Many colleagues have read multiple versions of the manuscript. In the UK, I thank Sari Wastell, Roger Sansi-Roca, Victoria Goddard, and Chris Wright for their constructive insights at different moments of this project. I am especially indebted to Frances Pine and Paola Filippucci for their close readings and advice. Parts of this manuscript were also read and commented upon by Ph.D. colleagues in London. I thank Aimee Joyce, Souad Osserain, Taras Fedirko, Akshi Singh, Katie Aston, Stephanie Grohman, Magdalena Buchczyck, Alexandra Urdea, Gabriela

Nicolescu, and William Tantam for their constant engagement and fruitful discussions. In Spain, I am grateful for the continuous feedback of Francisco Ferrándiz, who also allowed me to present parts of this research at the permanent seminar Faces and Traces of Violence at the Spanish National Research Council in March 2015. I also thank my colleagues Jorge Moreno Andrés and Lee Douglas for our long-term collaborations.

I am immensely indebted to my family and especially to my mother Maria and my grandmother Piedad for their optimism, fortitude and love. I am also forever grateful to my friends Clea House, Arturo Roura, Jo Kurukchi, Martina Larsson, Michael Vine, Cristina Gallardo, David Medja Fernández, Edu Cervera, and Antonio Gabás for listening to my ideas, reading some of the early drafts and supporting and encouraging this research throughout the years. Last, I thank the editors of this series, Emily Russell and Carmel Kennedy, for overseeing the publication of the manuscript and artist Ciara O'Brien for the illustration of the map of the region.

Geneva, Switzerland
April 2017

Contents

Acronyms and Abbreviations

AMECADEC	Association for the Memory of Castuera Concentration Camp
AMECECA (Previously PROMECECA)	Association for a Memorial in Cáceres Cemetery
ARMH	Association for the Recovery of Historical Memory
ARMHEx	Association for the Recovery of Historical Memory in Extremadura
CGT	General Confederation of Labour
El Foro	Forum for Memory
GEHCEx	Contemporary History Research Group in Extremadura
IU	United Left
PNV	Basque Nationalist Party
PP	Popular Party
PREMHEx	Project for the Recovery of Historical Memory
PSOE	Spanish Socialist Workers' Party
UGT	General Workers' Union
UN	United Nations
WGEID	Working Group on Enforced or Involuntary Disappearance

List of Figures

CHAPTER 1

The Archive, the Story and the Mass Grave

This book is a study of the impact that the exhumation of mass graves from the Spanish Civil War (1936–1939) has had on the understanding of the conflict in present day Extremadura, the region where I come from in southwestern Spain. When I began this research, I was clueless about many of the stories and sites, objects and archives that I would encounter later on, which revealed details about a history of victory and defeat that had rarely been shared between those I knew when growing up. The history of the Civil War was indeed never part of conversations at home, among friends or even, at school. The conflict seemed to exist in a distant yet present manner in my immediate surroundings. Many of the most intimate stories about the war, it would become clear to me with time and through this study, had remained part of personal exchanges often transmitted, as anthropologist Francisco Ferrándiz (2006) has poignantly put it, through cries and whispers. Many of these accounts, especially those connected to the losing side of the war, had remained outside of public and political debates during the Franco regime (1939–1975) and during the transition to democracy, which started in 1975. The memory of the war became an uncomfortable memory for many years, which had rarely found a space in social dialogue, history textbooks or other media reports at large.

The opening of a mass grave, in the year 2000, containing the human remains of left-wing Republicans killed by Francoist army members and supporters in the village of Priaranza del Bierzo in 1936 would return

Z. Aragüete-Toribio, *Producing History in Spanish Civil War Exhumations*, World Histories of Crime, Culture and Violence,
DOI 10.1007/978-3-319-61270-6_1

these stories and memories to the public realm more than six decades after the conflict had taken place. Though historians in academic circles had written much about the conflict since the end of the dictatorship (Juliá 2006, 2010), this exhumation sparked a process of historical inquiry into past Francoist crimes, which developed hand in hand with a strong campaign for the official recognition of such violent events. Mass graves evoked the unfinished reparation of the defeated and their silent histories of loss. They also became proof of one of the most uncharted forms of repression during the conflict: that of the extrajudicial detention, imprisonment and killing of Republicans, whose deaths were never atoned and whose corpses were never recovered after the war. When I began my research, I went back to the place where I grew up, Extremadura, where I encountered the trails of these events in people's stories and in the writing of historians, in kin-related narratives of violence and in the archaeological records of the mass-grave scientific interventions in which I worked.

As I began my research I was inspired by the way in which families, activists, scientists and historians had come together in the search for clues about the whereabouts of those in mass graves and their uncertain histories of death, which had mostly remained unspoken between different generations. As I arrived in Extremadura for a short summer visit, I was eager to learn firsthand what had happened to those who won but especially those who lost the war. In a pilot project in 2010, I established a first contact with some of the relatives and associations with whom I would work later on, hearing snippets of these traumatic stories and how people, in return, remembered and got to know about them. My newfound will to learn about this past, however, also led me to search for information within my own family, in an effort to understand how the people I knew related to the memory of the war and how silence had been established in a context that was familiar to me. That summer, I spoke to my grandmother about the things she remembered from the war. I was surprised to find out that, though she had never mentioned the subject at home, she seemed ready to retell to me the frail stories she could recall from those who were most affected by the conflict in the family.

My grandmother's account, a combination of firsthand and inherited memories, unveiled details about a story that neither my mother, my uncles, nor I had heard until that moment. The conversations with my grandmother were filled with anecdotes about three of her uncles—Felix,

Juan, and Casimiro—all of whom had fought in the Republican and Francoist armies throughout the conflict. In her account, she spoke about the way in which the three men underwent the threats and hardship of war. She recalled, for instance, how the youngest brother Felix had served in the Republican army in Madrid and was severely injured when he attempted to join the Francoist side. She also explained how Juan, the middle sibling, survived the war in Cádiz, where he had completed his military career—but how he later spent his last years in a psychiatric hospital, where he would die. Most poignantly, she recalled the death of Casimiro, the eldest of the three men, who was killed in Cataluña, where he had lived and worked as a member of the Republican military forces.

I was quickly taken by the story of Casimiro's death, which remained fuzzy and unclear in my grandmother's words. Though she had learnt about his demise from her mother and her aunts when growing up, she also recognized that the family never spoke openly about what happened to him. She could only tell me he had been killed in an ambush, together with ten other members of his regiment. According to her, the family never recovered the body. Its location and burial remained always unknown. Wanting to delve deeper into the fate of my distant and unfamiliar relative, my grandmother directed me to the confined space of a fragmented familial archive of letters and photographs, which one of her sisters had kept since the 1990s. These letters were part of the correspondence that her uncles exchanged with one another and with their parents during the years of their military service and around the time of the war. As I searched for information about my long-dead relatives, I began to acknowledge the piecemeal character of this historical research into such an elusive war past, as the testimony of my grandmother guided me to the writings of her uncles and to other family memorabilia, which unveiled the intimate stories of these three men.

In 2010, I collected numerous letters from my grandmother's sister's house with the hope to find hints about Casimiro's death. There was something impelling about these old and worn out documents, their inscriptions, and, in particular, the handwriting contained within them. As I read through the more than fifty letters, I unveiled a past that was foreign to me, but which felt, strangely, part of who I was. Each letter revealed some communication between my great-grandfather's brothers and the family over a period of two decades, from 1920 to 1939, speaking in detail about the everyday life in the military for my grandmother's uncles, and giving news of their parents from home. I felt impatient as I went through them. I examined each letter carefully, looking for information that hinted at the social tensions lived during the period that preceded the war. Letters dated 1935 already elucidated the agitated mood in the army and on the streets, but there were only a few of them. Following this, I could not find any letters written between 1935 and 1939. This unequivocal silence and rupture in their communication bitterly conveyed the outbreak of the war.

I had lost all hope of finding new information about Casimiro's death when, in the bundle of documents, I found a letter sent from the Catalan city of Mataró on the 15th March 1939 and addressed to my great-great grandparents. I was dumbfounded. The letter came from Casimiro's wife, Apolonia Martinez (see Fig. 1.1). In it, Apolonia described the events that took place before her husband's disappearance. She spoke about a quarrel Casimiro had had with a Republican corporal and how he felt threatened in his cadre after he was accused of "being a fascist." According to Apolonia, one of Casimiro's peers, Salvador, and he decided to join the Francoist army in a move to save their lives. Apolonia does not provide any other information about the clash Casimiro had with the corporal. Following her account, though, the incident appeared to me to be an ideological strife in the climate of suspicion and mistrust that must have reigned over the convoluted end of the war. Certainly, my grandmother had spoken to me, on many occasions, about the right-wing ideas shared by all members of her father's family. I wondered whether Francoist or in fact Republican forces had killed Casimiro. And so did Apolonia. Her letter, framed by the black edges that symbolized the mourning of a dead relative at the time, unfolded the frustration caused by the uncertainty that surrounded her husband's death. In an effort to clarify the circumstances of his disappearance, Apolonia asked Casimiro's parents—my great-great grandparents—to help her to elucidate what happened to him. In despair, she summoned them to inquire about his whereabouts:

> They gave him up for disappeared here [in Mataró] and I hoped you could investigate whether the nationalists [sic] captured him. I regret my luck but would not like his death to fall into obscurity. As it is the only thing I can do, I organized a mass for him and Salvador yesterday.

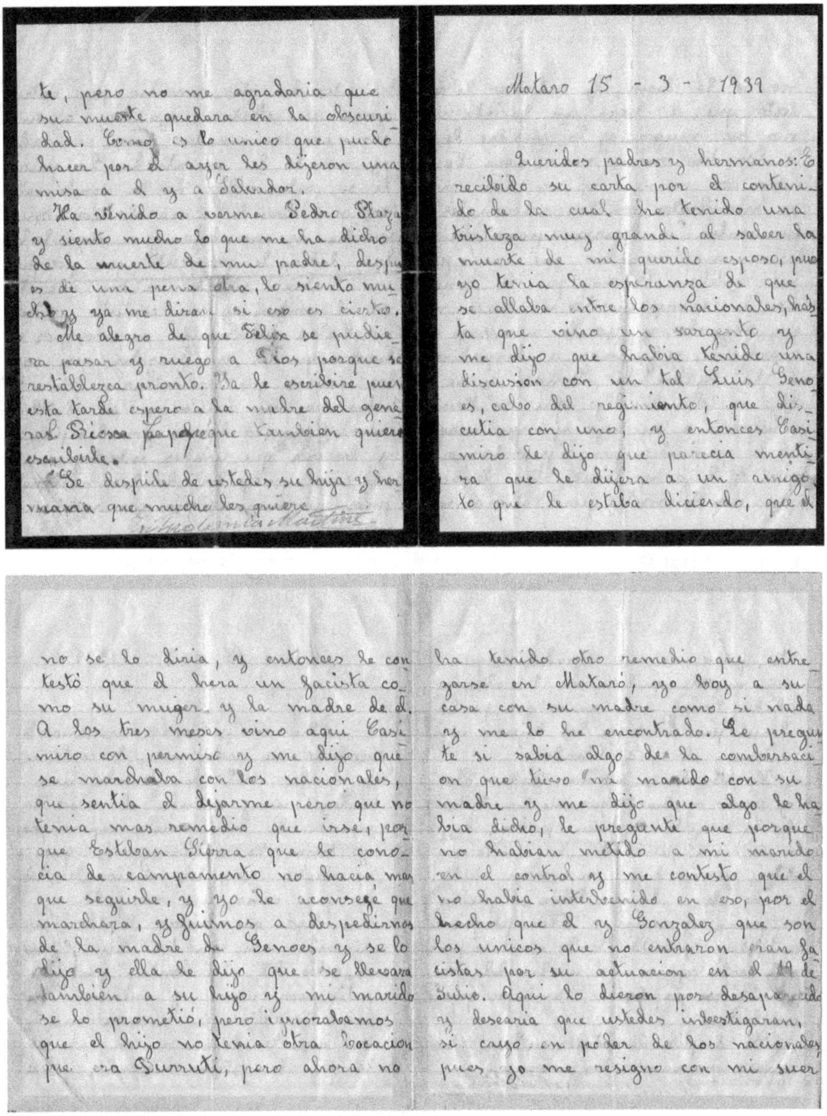

Mataro 15 - 3 - 1939

Queridos padres y hermanos: E recibido su carta por el contenido de la cual he tenido una tristeza muy grande al saber la muerte de mi querido esposo, pues yo tenia la esperanza de que se allaba entre los nacionales, hasta que vino un sargento y me dijo que habia tenido una discusion con un tal Luis Genoes, cabo del regimiento, que discutia con uno, y entonces Casimiro le dijo que parecia mentira que le dijera a un amigo lo que le estaba diciendo, que el

no se lo diria, y entonces le contestó que el hera un facista como su muger y la madre de el. A los tres meses vino aqui Casimiro con permiso y me dijo que se marchaba con los nacionales, que sentia el dejarme pero que no tenia mas remedio que irse, porque Esteban Sierra que le conocia de campamento no hacia mas que seguirle, y yo le aconsegé que marchara, y fuimos a despedirnos de la madre de Genoes y se lo dijo y ella le dijo que se llevara tambien a su hijo y mi marido se lo prometió, pero ignorabamos que el hijo no tenia otra bocacion que era Durruti, pero ahora no

ha tenido otro remedio que entregarse en Mataró, yo voy a su casa con su madre como si nada y me lo he encontrado. Le pregunte si sabia algo de la combersacion que tuvo mi marido con su madre y me dijo que algo le habia dicho, le pregunté que porque no habian metido a mi marido en el control y me contesto que el no habia intervenido en eso, por el hecho que el y Gonzalez que son los unicos que no entraron eran fascistas por su actuacion en el 19 de Julio. Aqui lo dieron por desaparecido y desearia que ustedes investigaran, si cayo en poder de los nacionales, pues yo me resigno con mi suer

te, pero no me agradaria que su muerte quedara en la obscuridad. Como es lo unico que puedo hacer por el ayer les dijeron una misa a el y a Salvador.

Ha venido a verme Pedro Plaza y siento mucho lo que me ha dicho de la muerte de mi padre, despues de una pena otra, lo siento mucho y ya me diran si eso es cierto.

Me alegro de que Felix se pudiera pasar y ruego a Dios porque se restablezca pronto. Ya le escribire pues esta tarde espero a la madre del general Riosca porque tambien quiere escribirle.

Se despide de ustedes su hija y hermana que mucho les quiere

Apolonia Martinez

Fig. 1.1 Letter from Apolonia Martinez describing the details of her husband's Casimiro disappearance, dated 15th March 1939

After reading the letter, I showed it to my grandmother and asked her if her grandparents had done anything about this. She was equally surprised, for she had not known about the document. "I think they did nothing," she reflected. She believed Casimiro's mother's illness and the lack of resources of the family in Extremadura made any search for her uncle at the end of the war improbable. Whether my great-great grandparents ever helped Apolonia, or even how they found out about Casimiro's death, would remain a mystery to me. It was then that I realized that there was information about my past—part of a broader national past—that I was never going to know. The discovery of the letter also struck my mother and some of her siblings, who had never been aware of such correspondence or the existence of these family members. When I took the letter back to my grandmother's house, my mother, she, and I read it together and listened to the memories that the document evoked for my grandmother. I recorded our voices as we read over Apolonia's words. I recorded them time and time again as we tried to decipher her particular handwriting and those expressions that, product by a different time, were peculiar to us. The letter, most certainly, came to represent an uncanny shared history and made us witnesses of Apolonia's distressing experience. By recording our voices, I aimed to produce a document of this intimate intergenerational moment, in which the three of us became connected to the Civil War past.

The experience with my family letters made me reflect, once again, on the experience of those who searched for the whereabouts of their long-gone kin in mass graves but also in the array of official documents, personal memorabilia, newspaper clippings, in narratives of survivors and in the pages of historians' books. The experience within my own family's archive made me think, then, about the potential for material and narrated fragments to activate the imagination and produce a personal yet public history of loss in the present. As the traces that evoked the fate of Casimiro inside the decaying personal repository elucidated, such remnants helped to sketch the contours of an absence—linked to the act of the execution and disappearance—which deeply marked the lives of distinct generations. I wondered about the force that these encounters exerted on the articulation of a wider historical narrative and on the shaping of new social, political and familial identities, connected to the recognition of such violent crimes. Through the finding of these letters, I uncovered the traces of an unspoken family past. In a similar manner, I considered how the encounter with the human remains, the testimony and the files that have emerged since the first exhumations of the twenty-first century occurred—and their relation to different forms of expertise—have created new forms of enunciation that speak to long-established historical discourses and different memory politics connected to the conflict. Such artefacts and their conceptualisation, I thought, transformed those who became involved in the process and also the ways in which the past has come to be known in recent years.

History Between the Archive and the Grave

From the beginning of my research in Extremadura, I became interested in the forms of information gathering that had taken place around the exhumation of human remains buried in Civil War mass graves. In the region, this process was deeply entangled with the investigation that an ample group of historians inside and outside of the regional university had started even before exhumations occurred. One could say, however, as pointed out in the next chapters, that the search for the Republican killed accelerated these scientific explorations into the past, which, in Extremadura, focused especially on the study of episodes of extrajudicial repression—such as clandestine executions—or judicial processes that gave place to hundreds of summary executions and thousands of life-long prison sentences. When I began my research in Extremadura, there was also a public interest in other episodes of past Francoist violence against Republican women during and after conflict; against Republican prisoners in Camps, prisons and work battalions; and against the Republican families who survived into the years of the Franco regime.

One of the most active teams that engaged with the subject of Francoist repression in the region was the institutional Project for the Recovery of Historical Memory in Extremadura (*Proyecto para la Recuperación de la Memoria Histórica en Extremadura* or PREMHEx), which was funded by the regional administration and hosted by the History Department in the University of Extremadura. The project, born out of a political and scientific will to investigate the experience of Republican defeat in the region, drew from the examination of official archives in military repositories and civil registries, the collection of testimonies from relatives and survivors, and the exhumation of mass graves. When I approached the field, I became fascinated by the amount of information that the project had amassed but also by the efforts that its researchers—together with other independent historians, activists, relatives of those killed during the conflict, and survivors—made to reunite distinct documentation and oral accounts to cross-reference and contest the data in the Francoist archive.

Such a process of association, as one could call it, was driven by a will to provide an alternative vision of the conflict, which repositioned Francoist official sources and spoke to its silences and euphemisms with counter-stories that retold Republican experiences of death, persecution and deprivation. During my stay in Extremadura, I observed that these official archives were the source against which the search for, location and identification of corpses occurred. The absence of full details about the killings of the defeated in Francoist files and historiography was representative of the types of facts and taxonomic order that the Franco regime imposed after the war ended. Speaking of how historical works have represented different struggles in the Haitian revolution, Michel-Rolph Trouillot (1995, 52) has observed the selective work that takes place in the creation of new archives and how power imbalances that exist outside of these repositories determine the management, organization and writing of their content. In Spain, new processes of classification enabled the New State or *Nuevo Estado*—as Francoist authorities would call it—to provide a chronicle of the victory of the war, creating new categories attached to the so-called Republican enemy. The regime's archival collections also set, as Trouillot (ibid.) observed in his own work, the "conditions" for the existence of some statements and not others; of that which could be said and that which had to be silenced. The official archive was, evoking the author's words, also in Spain, an instutionalized site that "convey[ed] authority and set the rules of credibility and interdependence, help[ing] to select the stories that matter[ed]" (ibid., 52). Description and reference inside the Spanish postwar archive were subject to Franco's desire for domination and the exclusion of the left-wing from the emerging political and social milieu, and the national historical narrative.

Many of the people I worked with during fieldwork, engaged with a definition of these official archives as deceitful. They understood the depictions of left-wing Republicans as false or distorted by the intentions of Francoist authorities. This view of the official archive recognizes a power asymmetry at play in the incorporation of information to the repository. It further denounces the information they contain and the military and judicial processes they speak of, placing its files at the centre of contemporary social claims for recognition. Other anthropological studies (see Trundle

2011; Murphy 2011; Kaplonski 2011) have shown how state documents become sources that confront families and civil society groups vis-à-vis the state, and are redefined in the context of their search for legitimacy. Files might stand as unknown remainders of a traumatic personal history that reveal new information about an intimate past upon being encountered (Murphy 2011). They might also be proof of fatal events or past repression in endeavours for compensation or rehabilitation in the face of reluctant administrations (Trundle 2011; Kaplonski 2011). Moreover, these and other works highlight the relational character of these sources, as their social meanings are entangled with the existence of other people, sites and documents that provide alternative forms of witnessing and re-interpret the logic of the archive. On her work on the files of re-settlement programmes during the Indian Emergency period, Emma Tarlo (2003, 9) has likewise observed that state documents are of anthropological interest not only for their "content but also for the circumstances surrounding their production, circulation and interpretation". In Spain, thinking about military and historical files means to enter in contact with the families, activists and historians that often seek to mend the power inequalities that produced them, by explaining its form and content in connection to the information that emerges from the exhumation process.

The search for the Republicans buried in mass graves triggered new forms of collecting that have put official files in contact with other artefacts such as familial objects, letters, biographical sketches, family images, historical writings or scientific reports about the human remains in mass burials. Conversely, writing about a particular exhumation project in Castilla La Mancha, Spain, anthropologist Lee Douglas (2014) has also spoken about the labour of contextualisation that takes place at the grave, as forensic evidence is always analysed in conjunction with other artefacts, state documents and personal testimonies. The search for those in mass graves often involves the location of their names in civil registries, the compilation of names absent in the archive from the stories of those who knew how acts of extrajudicial repression took place, and the final scientific investigation of these killings—which often unveiled new facts about the people who were murdered and the act of the execution. As Douglas (2014, 5) has observed "there is not a unique starting point for this chain of knowledge collection and production. The relationship between diverse knowledge forms is symbiotic, malleable and changing." The process hence revealed itself as multidirectional. It occurred from the archive into the grave and from the grave into other private and public milieux. Official archives, human remains, personal objects and documents, and life histories hence, became intrinsic to such knowledge assemblages, prompting new forms of circulation and acts of cross-examination, comparison, and substantiation that aimed to resolve long-standing uncertainties about the killings.

Absence, as Lee Douglas (2014) has also observed, is a defining aspect of the location and exhumation of human remains in Spain. Absences permeated the official archive—in the inconsistent and patchy information, which resulted from the omission of records or the disappearance of files in the aftermath of the war and dictatorship. They also imbued individual and community memories, as silence and fear had also damaged the social transmission of these events across generations. Extrajudicial killings, which were often referred to as *sacas* or *paseos*—literary meaning to take someone out or to take someone for a walk—happened in the middle of the night or at dawn, in the middle of the countryside, in roadsides or at the rear of municipal cemeteries. Sometimes these killings left witnesses, which had voluntarily or forcibly attended the executions. In most cases, rumours pervaded the communities where they occurred, making the event subject to manifold ambiguities. In the archive, their record, if it existed, was often deferred, made months or even years after the killings had taken place. The search for and exhumation of the corpses of victims of these executions has revealed, as will be explored throughout the book, intense acts of "figuring out" in the present through incessant conversations, scientific and historical analyses and exchanges among the living. In these acts, the materiality of the conflict, its "traces"—as Antoine Prost (2001) might refer to them—became not only vehicles but also agents (Latour 1999) in the production of new meanings connected to the repressive act and in the transformation of a social milieu where new claims could be uttered.

In these performances, these acts of collection and recollection, these instances of "figuring out," which were part and parcel of the exhumation process, the concept of the archive became once again alive in my research. Nevertheless, this time, its image was not so much connected to the repository housed in the institution, as Trouillot (1995) had understood it—though there were fragments from these registers too. The archive presented itself as a multi-sited entity that encompassed new techniques for knowing the past and epistemic sites of production and interpretation in which the encounter with material and oral remnants generated other idioms, other conversations, other discourses—which have become gradually more established throughout the last decade—in relation to the rights and the state recognition of those who had suffered the violence of the war and the dictatorship.

In this book, I entertain two principal notions of the archive that are in constant interaction with and inform one another. One vision of the archive is directly connected to its physical presence as a site of state production; to its buildings and rooms; to its registers and its records of bureaucratic activity that are distributed, classified and processed according to particular documentation and archivization protocols. This is the space where administrative, historical and military files live and one of the places that the historian visits more frequently. Whereas this study contemplates the archive as institutional space, it does not do so with the intention to examine in detail the way in which state archival collections are organized, catalogued or indexed, for example. The book touches upon these themes insomuch as the management and especially the access to such sources condition and are intrinsic to the experience of researching history in the archive. Following the work of historians such as Carolyn Steedman (2001a, b), I explore the labour of the historian in the archive and with state documents, and also pay special attention to the way in which other groups relate to these files once they are circulated in the public realm. In *Dust* (2001b) and some of her preceding essays, Steedman foregrounds the concreteness of the archive as a necessary site where historical study begins. In opposition to other works such as Derrida's (1996) seminal lecture, later turned into a book, *Archive Fever*, Steedman argues for an understanding of the source that takes into account the effects and affective capacity of its materiality over those who research it.

Steedman critiques the metaphoric meaning that Derrida provides to the archive in his exploration of Freud's collection of letters, writings and notes. Derrida's notion emerges from a will to understand how psychoanalysis came into being, and is particularly concerned with the process of *archivization* through which information is selected, discarded, or destroyed to compose Freud's archive as we know it today. Evoking Freud's psychoanalytic preoccupations, Derrida (ibid., 14) identifies destruction as the "vocation" of the archive, as the drive that guides the making of the source: these are acts that move its creator to efface, forget or silence his or her own "traces". This is what Derrida calls the death drive of archival activity. Such tendency is, moreover, in constant tension with yet another impulse to seek, collect and preserve information, with a desire for conservation. It is this double bind that generates what the writer calls the *mal d'archive* or which provides such feverish and unsettling quality to the archive itself. In the context of this book, I have interpreted such a *mal d'archive*, which is at times invoked throughout the work, in relation to the incessant and burning searches that people perform inside and outside the official archive in order to compile an assemblage of traces that surpassed imposed silences and resisted unresolved gaps in national and personal historical narratives. I use the expression, however, also in the way Carolyn Steedman (2001a) has used it in her commentary of Derrida's text. Claiming a more experiential approach to the archive, Steedman (2001a) has described *archive fever* as the sickness and bodily discomfort, as the disease that the archive causes among those who touch its ledgers and breathe its dust. I draw from this phenomenological vision of the archive and expand on it to include the reactions, torments, anxiety and angst that the act of searching, deciphering and interpreting the archive often prompted in those who looked for clues in official files, in personal collections and in new scientific registers about unresolved extrajudicial killings. I am interested here in how the archive is internalized and somatised as well as on how it *feels*.

A second view engages with a broad definition that sees the archive as a wide-raging process of classification, ordering and production of statements that is enabled by certain conditions of possibility. This vision is connected to Michel Foucault's (1972) notion of the archive in his *Archaeology of Knowledge*. In Foucault's theoretical work, the archive is the system through which statements come into being and which differentiates the contours of distinct discourses. One could interpret, as I propose in this study, the understanding of the exhumation process in this sense, as a developing alternative archive that has transformed the discourse of history through the emergence of new accounts or statements of scientific, social and political order. As such, and following other anthropological works that have considered the archive as process (Stoler 2002, 2009; Edwards 2014), I explore the exhumation archive in connection to the social relations that engender it, which expand the temporal dimension of diverse generations; to the power dynamics that shape its forms of production, notation, accumulation, and analysis; to the uncertainties and anxieties that confound the process; and to the type of knowledge they author as well as its place in convoluted and competing historical discourses. Throughout an ethnographic journey that begins with the historian's work and archive—in itself an assemblage of objects from many other repositories—and continues at the mass grave (where other materials converge) I explore the structure and method of the archiving process but also what Stoler (2009) has termed as its "pulse" or affective force.

This conceptual metaphor has influenced my own methodology. Drawing on the expansive quality that such metaphor affords (Marcus 1995), I aimed to trace the contours of such an archive by following the trajectory of human remains and the stories that surrounded them, through different sites of knowledge exchange—following the people, spaces, and things that took part in such process of epistemological transmission. It required to adopt what George Marcus (1995) once termed as a multi-sited approach to fieldwork that would lead me to commemorative acts and book launches, political meetings and interviews with associations members, history books, exhibitions, laboratory work, exhumation campaigns, round tables and conferences, summer courses, and the manifold private and public spaces where families moved and retold their intimate stories of violence. Material objects, paper files and human remains became a central element of this network that would construct and delimit the field as I understand it in this work (Coleman and Collins 2006).

During the first months in Extremadura, in 2011, I conducted interviews with activists, historians and some relatives, and attended numerous events that happened in springtime around the anniversary of the start of the Second Republic on 14th April 1931. My focus shifted to the exhumation site as I was invited to participate in an excavation in the village of Castuera (Badajoz) by PREMHEx archaeologist Laura Muñoz-Encinar and the president of the association who promoted the intervention (see Chap. 4). In the summer of 2012, I would work at two more sites, namely, Puebla de Alcocer and Fregenal de la Sierra (Badajoz), with a team led by the same archaeologist (see Chap. 5). In these different locations, I worked jointly with the scientific team, in and outside of the mass grave; I conversed with groups of families, activists, and neighbours; and I followed the work of local historians. At the site, I was able to track life histories, scientific interpretations, and historical work, and to observe how people related to human remains and their objects. It also allowed me to follow objects into other places such as family and historians' homes that provided intimate meanings to the objects that guided our conversations and to the information that was shared. Being at the heart of this process allowed me to trace connections that extended in time and space. It also enabled me to examine the situated knowledge and experience of different subjects, especially in relation to three evidentiary traces, namely, the corpse, the testimony and the state document.

Following the Exhumation Archive and its Evidentiary Traces

As in other contexts worldwide (see Kwon 2006; Petrović-Šteger 2008; Wagner 2008; Sanford 2003; Crossland 2013), unmarked mass graves in Spain pointed to the unceremonial burial of human remains, the absence of any public remembrance, and the impossibility of familial mourning and commemoration after conflict—and throughout decades. The exhumation campaign in Spain has happened in a context of international debates and practices around the rights of victims of extreme violence and in the framework of transitional justice initiatives that have been implemented worldwide since the 1980s. Scholars in social and forensic anthropology, law, history or political science (Ferrádiz 2014; Gatti 2016; Ferrándiz and Robben 2015; Garibian 2015; Fondebrider 2015b; Kovras 2014; Crossland 2013; Rojas-Pérez 2015; Rubin 2014) have discussed how exhumations are part of other truth-seeking mechanisms developed in connection to "the global expansion of international human rights discourses and its accompanying institutions and practices, as well as to a parallel and equally transnational trend to display, commemorate, and memorialise atrocities" (Ferrándiz and Robben 2015, 7). Some of these transnational endeavours have surfaced from grassroots' appeals in relation to human rights violations and crimes against humanity committed during wars or authoritarian regimes (ibid.). A case in point, and possibly one of the most significant to the expansion of such legal, political and social paradigm worldwide is that of Argentina, where, after intense social campaigning for the search of thousands of people who disappeared during the government of the military junta (1976–1983), exhumations and truth trials began to take place (Garibian 2015; Gatti 2016; Fondebrider 2015b).

In these transitional justice processes, which have often been guided by the tenets of liberal democracy (Teitel 2000, 2003; Golob 2008; Kovras 2014), particular "truth-seeking" strategies have been deployed as fundamental tools to guarantee the reparation of past crimes and their non-repetition. In these contexts, work with human remains, testimonies, and documents from state archives and beyond has been part of exhumations, truth and reconciliation commissions, trials or commemorative projects aimed at discerning a "truthful" account of the causes and effects of past violence. Such investigations have involved the work of experts but also the collaboration of witnesses, relatives of the victims, perpetrators and grassroots organizations, among others, that have provided specific meanings to such materiality of conflict. In relation to the corpses buried in mass graves that result from extrajudicial executions and other forms of violent repression, forensic work has helped to document and prosecute gross human rights violations—through the aid of scientific methods (Ferrándiz and Robben 2015; Rosenblatt 2015; Crossland 2013; Crossland and Joyce 2015; Dreyfus and Anstett 2015; Congram 2016; Wagner 2008). Forensic expertise has been used in post-conflict judicial proceedings since the aftermath of World War II (Ferrándiz and Robben 2015). Most recently, two of the most influential tribunals of the last decades, namely, the International Criminal Tribunal for the Former Yugoslavia, created in 1993, and the International Criminal Tribunal for Rwanda, created in 1994, have relied, as Ferrándiz and Robben (ibid., 10) have stated, on scientific finds and reports from exhumations to aid their verdicts.

Nevertheless, current inquiries into past human rights violations have transformed the nature, definition and practice of forensic work, understood traditionally as a type of scientific labour associated with legal prosecution and the realm of the courtroom (Fondebrider 2015a; Rosenblatt 2015). Forensic anthropologist Luis Fondebrider (2015a) has advocated for a holistic understanding of the work of the forensic expert—a category which might encompass forensic anthropologists and archaeologists—in post-conflict international investigations. This approach involves a consideration of other humanitarian meanings to their work, as their endeavours also include the return of the dead to their living family or the mediation of conflict among civil society actors, often, in politically complex domains. In a similar manner, Adam Rosenblatt (2015, 13) ascertains that "the very idea of the 'forensic' has undergone a profound shift" in the last decades, as forensic work has diversified and began to expand into other investigative areas of violence. Like Fondebrider, the author also observes that such a shift is determined by the role that forensic experts have acquired as intermediaries between international requirements and local cultural views around the unearthing and treatment of the dead. This, in the words of Rosenblatt (ibid.), has presented forensic investigations with "extraordinary political and ethical challenges", as scientists contend with the novelty and contingency that each post-violence setting encompasses. Human remains, objects, testimonies and a diversity of state and non-state documents have become intrinsic to the epistemology and labours of recent forensic inquiries into human rights violations, becoming nods that elucidate the specific scientific approaches, conceptualisations and skills that emerge in radically distinct post-repression sites.

In this study, I approach these three traces in exhumation projects that take place in a context in which human remains, testimonies and distinct files hold no legal status as part court proceedings or judicial investigations. Most local and national judges in Spain have expressed an unwillingness to probe into past Civil War and postwar killings basing their decision on the restrictions imposed by the Amnesty Law that has existed in the country since 1977, as discussed in Chap. 2. As a result, post-transitional initiatives (Aguilar 2008) such as exhumations, which have been led mostly by civil society groups, have aimed, on the one hand, to alleviate and recognize publically the suffering of families and survivors affected by Francoist violence and, on the other, to compile information about these crimes. Though there has not been much of a concerted effort on the part of state institutions to regulate exhumation practice in Spain (only one state protocol has been issued since these scientific endeavours began in the year 2000), the diversity of archaeological teams that have emerged to conduct these interventions around the country have, more often than not, worked with a purpose to document mass grave excavations following international forensic standards in the investigation of human rights abuses. They have done so with a humanitarian intention to search and identify victims but also with a goal to generate reports about past mass crimes that can be used in possible future prosecution proceedings or in a truth commission.

The work on mass graves led by the archaeologists that I collaborated with in Extremadura resembled, as forensic anthropologist Hugh Tuller (2015) has observed in other contexts, the labour of investigators at a crime scene. Both groups of professionals Tuller (ibid., 94) argues "use many of the same tools and processes to tease out and record relevant information from a site." Both also, according to the author (ibid.), "adhere to the same mantra: you only get one chance to get it right." Archaeologists and crime scene investigators both pay detailed attention to the contextual information that can be obtained about an event and use methods that maximise data retrieval in such a destructive investigative process. In this regard, throughout the book, I refer to the scientific work carried out at the mass grave as archaeogical, as human remains were studied to interpret the historical acts of violence that produced such killings, and that could be inferred from the marks on the skeletons and their disposition in the burial pit. I also refer to archaeological labour as forensic, for, even outside of the framework of a judicial inquiry, such work entailed acts of observation, and recording and documentation adapted to particular protocols and driven by the will to turn these corpses in mass graves into what Rojas-Pérez (2015) has described as "legal subjects" through the institutionalization of such inquiries. Scientists with whom I worked sought to provide proof of the intentionality behind Franco's repressive campaign and the systematic character of the crimes—something that spoke directly to the notion of "crime against humanity" enshrined in international human rights law. They also aimed to create new "historical subjects" (ibid.), as the information produced at the mass grave also became part of historical studies (Crossland 2013) in the region about the idiosyncrasies of war and postwar violence and the number of Republican victims.

In the exhumations I followed, human remains, testimonies and different archival documents acquired a relational character as indexes that pointed to the forms of terror lived at the sites that scientists excavated. Speaking about a particular exhumation project in the area of Ayacucho, Peru, Isaias Rojas Pérez (2015, 41) has observed how the work of forensic scientists, with whom he worked in the search for various mass burials containing the bodies of victims of the counterinsurgency campaigns of the 1980s and 1990s, was intrinsically connected to what Carlo Ginzburg identifies as the "epistemology of the clue." This is, according to the author, "the idea that a trained and detached observer is able to read the clues and traces left by the past as means of gaining otherwise inaccessible truths." In Peru, Rojas-Pérez (2015) argues that such scientific practice is intimately entangled with the work of the law and thus influenced by its controlled language and procedures. The author demonstrates, however, how research into the workings of past terror brings these epistemic frameworks and strategies in tension, as the search for those executed is filled with contradictions and the appearance of often unexpected or contingent information (ibid.) challenges scientific and legal rationalizations. In his example, it is the voice of an unknown witness of the crimes that challenges the method and interpretation of scientific and legal work, as it resolves some of the ambivalence that exists around the acts of killing and burial that took place in the locality. In a similar manner, Chaps. 3, 4 and 5 of this book deal with how the method of the historian, the archaeologist and the physical anthropologist conversed with the complex manifestation of personal experiences of the conflict that occurred in the villages where mass graves were located and exhumed. On the one hand, community narratives often challenged the understanding that scientists had of these traces. On the other, such clues and their scientific interpretation also destabilized long-established community perceptions of the killings. At the heart of the analysis, I posit a reflection on how the uncertainty generated by violence (also in Rojas-Pérez 2015) and its temporal replay across generations shapes the interaction between different modes of knowledge production at the exhumation site.

Human remains are thus at the centre of scientific examinations performed through the dictums of "objectivity" and "detachment" (Renshaw 2011, 156) that govern scientific practice and which often aim to generate concrete and fixed understandings of the past (see also Rojas-Pérez). Nevertheless, as Rojas-Pérez (2015) but also other authors like Joyce (2015), Rosenblatt (2015), Fondebrider (2015a, b), Crossland (2013), Renshaw (2011) or Wagner (2008) have demonstrated in other contexts, this does not mean to say that scientific work is completely neutral or that bones are mere artefacts through which to discern unmediated truths. As forensic expert Francisco Etxeberría (2012), and also Crossland and Joyce (2015) have implied, scientists that work on the investigation of human rights violations have a social commitment. Moreover, Layla Renshaw (2011) has widely discussed in her own study of exhumations of Civil War mass graves in northern

Spain how archaeologists and forensic experts negotiated the demands for impartiality and detachment that their own discipline and training instilled in them, with the inadvertent emotional responses that the presence of tortured, abused and maltreated corpses produced in them. The author describes moments in which archaeologists identify personally with those in the grave, as some of the objects that appeared next to the bodies, their possessions, revealed shared habits between the living and the dead. In other instances, Renshaw depicts the way in which expert practitioners imagined the person, to whom a skeleton belonged in life, through the amalgam of information that circulates in the space of the exhumation. The author retells how, in these moments, expressions of compassion and sorrow for the suffering of the victims were often uttered, highlighting the idea that the labour of excavating these human remains was also an intimate and affective undertaking. Renshaw's (ibid., 184) argument concludes that, at the exhumation site, "the materialisation of the dead through their bodies and objects elicited powerful emotions and afforded a complex range of representations." Human remains in these contexts are more than just artefacts or things. They are, above all, a part of someone that once was and as such, they evoke, as Rojas-Pérez (2015, 56) has stated, a person "with a set of social relations".

The exposure of these skeletons prompted the imagination of the victims for scientists at the site but also animated the retelling of witness' accounts that aimed to sketch a portrait of those buried and of the act of execution. Within the space of the mass grave, stories proliferated, moving seamlessly between different periods of the past and the present, retelling the event of the killings, the episodes that preceded it and the experience of postwar repression that many endured thereafter. On many occasions, families, neighbours and onlookers gathered around the dig attempting to define a common narrative of the event, reacting to finds in the grave or to the information shared by scientists. Other moments, accounts were provided for the purpose of scientific pre-mortem studies, historical analysis or anthropological inquiry in more structured or semi-structured interviews—which sometimes resembled a witness deposition. Nevertheless, in the realm of the mass grave *life histories, accounts* or *stories*, as I will refer to them—depending on how they were told, their length and content—acquired a different pace, flexibility and open-ended character. These oral records became more like maps through which, as anthropologist Julie

Cruickshank (1998, 2) has stated, one could "establish connections—between past and future, between people and place, among people whose opinions diverge." In this book, there are parts of extended life histories and references to brief conversations, in one-to-one encounters or as part of a group, in and out the scenario of the mass grave. These stories, moreover, reflected the experiences of members of distinct generations: some were the children of those who died; others were their grandchildren—who had often been told little about what happened to their ancestors; others were the great-grandchildren—who often knew vaguely about these killings but who promoted vigorous searches for information in order to comprehend such complex and hidden family past. Such moments of retelling were social acts that attested collective experiences at the mass grave. These forms of storytelling also took place in more intimate spaces, such as the household, where individuals attempted to voice and recompose a biographical history fractured by political repression.

For many of the relatives of the victims, the memory of the killings remained fuzzy, for such events had hardly been shared among the members of different generations. Cultural theorists such as Astrid Erll (2011) or Jan Assmann (1995) have understood the family as a framework that enables the transfer of social and individual knowledge and experience through communicative and bodily acts between generations. In these familial exchanges, certain communicative structures have often become vehicles through which people narrate their pasts and experience, creating intimate bonds among kin. Marianne Hirsch (2008, 2012) has problematized the idea of mnemonic transmission within the family that some of these authors entertain by considering how disruptive events, such as war violence, transform these communicative structures within the family and affect the qualities of transmission. For Hirsch (2008, 209), who has widely researched how intergenerational acts of knowledge and memory transfer occurred among the generations that survived the Holocaust and their descendents, material fragments that remain such as photographs constitute objects of "remembrance that reconnect and re-embody an intergenerational memorial fabric that was severed by catastrophe." Chapter 6 pays special attention to these forms of familial remembrance in intimate yet shared spaces of testimony. On the one hand, it looks at how family voices attest individual experiences of violence (Das 2007). On the other, it focuses on the way people relate to traces that form new personal archives that have emerged as a result of exhumation processes. Death certificates, prison files, sentences from summary judgements, personal letters, photographs, old family books or biographical writings are used to re-assemble the memory of an unknown relative. This process, I will argue, is fraught with the same anxiety that also imbues the site of the exhumation. Abject sensations mark the encounter with the materiality of the past in these personal collections, as in state archives, for the effects of violence can still be traced in the texture, grain and messages that these objects contain (Hirsch 2012; Navaro-Yashin 2012).

The presence of the corpse—mediated through the expressions and vocabularies of scientific expertise (Crossland 2013; Rosenblatt 2015) and through other mnemonic articulations—along with the testimony and the files from state and other archives have indeed become forms of evidence "through the performative acts of exhumation, display and analysis" (Crossland and Joyce (2015, 4) that take place in the search for those who were killed in extrajudicial executions in Spain. The stories of these victims have proliferated from the space of the mass grave and the home to the arena of the public. Francisco Ferrándiz (2014) has explained how historical memory associations have invested great efforts to gather and communicate these accounts in media and digital realms. Accounts about past Francoist violence have become the basis for new forms of social activism and campaigns that seek to re-signify the identity of victims and the political community of the living. As in other contexts, the new representations and materialisations of the Civil War dead have emerged (Renshaw 2011), as the information produced has entered other channels of transmission that aimed to shape collective interpretations of the war whilst redefining the relation between individuals, communities and the state.

Reordering Individual and Collective Worlds

Recovering, identifying, and reburying the corpses of the Republican defeated are regarded as acts that dignify the memory of the deceased and restore their place both in history and in the social imaginary of the nation. As many scholars have discussed (Kovras 2014; Hayner 2011; Teitel 2000; Encarnación 2008) the search for truth has been a central tenet and a moral imperative (Kovras 2014) in order to achieve successful democratization through the rule of law. "Dealing with the past" has thus been seen by some scholars and practitioners as a crucial component to realize a kind of political and democratic stability after conflict (Wouters 2014; Bell 2009). It has also been central to institutional and political approaches to conflict and post-conflict forms of reconciliation. NGOs and organizations such as the United Nations (UN) have declared that "victims and their families have the imprescriptible right to know the truth about the circumstances in which violations took place and, in the event of death or disappearance, the victims' fate" (2005 UN report on impunity by Diane Orentlicher cited in Hayner 2011, 24). This right to the truth, which has been established as an obligation of states, is inevitably connected to the incorporation of particular histories of repression and violence to the country's collective memory.

Conversely, investigative processes into the past and the claims for truth that these might generate have been deployed to define the nature of past mass crimes in order to re-signify particular collective political identities in the present. In his work on Cyprus, Paul Sant Cassia (2005) has discussed how the articulation of distinct narratives of past violence about the losses suffered by both Greek and Turkish Cypriot communities during the conflict that expanded the decades of the 1960s and the 1970s, has aided to redefine the social boundaries of both groups in the Cypriot post-conflict milieu. Claims for distinct historical truths have incorporated the stories of the "missing" with a purpose to establish the contours of two emerging states after extreme political violence. In these exploits, Sant Cassia (ibid.) has explained that new categorizations of the dead have helped political actors in both groups but also victims realize claims about the past, present and future of both communities. As the author explains, the Greek community has often referred to those who went missing as a result of the Turkish invasion of 1974 as "disappeared," stating that these people, who were alive when they were captured, could still be alive at present. Arguing for the uncertainty and indefinite suffering that surviving families undergo, such categorization has allowed Greek groups to emphasize the ongoing character of the crimes committed by the Turkish state. Moreover, it has also internationalised their claim, as they appeal to international agencies in order to categorise these events in the international language of rights. By contrast, the Turkish Cypriot counterpart has classed those that went missing in the conflict, as "dead" in order to, according to the author, highlight the crimes committed by Greek groups and to distance themselves from their neighbouring community. Such victims' categorizations, the history of these events and the memories of survivors aid institutional actors in creating a particular vision and rhetoric for how the past should be remembered (Sant Cassia 2005, 25).

The absence of state involvement in civil society-led truth-seeking initiatives and the lack of trials—where, as Soshana Felman (2002) has observed, past silences in overarching historical discourses can be subverted through the enactment of private and collective traumas—has opened up an area for narrating the past that occurs on the margins of existing memory politics in Spain. When I arrived in Extremadura during fieldwork, I observed that remembering the past, as Michael Lambek (1996) has argued, had become an ethical and moral practice for many of these groups that drew on new symbolic representations and idioms in relation to the war dead to claim new political collectivites. As Lambek (1996, 239) observed in his work on memory and spirit possession in Madagascar, "the value of articulating a particular version of the past was [for these collectives], explicitly connected to its moral ends and consequences for relations in the present." Through the organization of different events, which ranged from demonstrations to commemorative acts, these civil society associations demanded "truth, justice and reparation," confronting the state head on and redefining human rights consciousness. In these new expressions, the notion of the "disappeared" has also played a vital role, as discussed in Chap. 2, becoming part of a new vocabulary that has translated individual experiences of ambiguity over a relative's death and the whereabouts of their corpse into global international human rights discourses. On the other, however, such denomination also encounters local manifestations connected to the complete disappearance of the body and of evidence from archives and other repositories, as pointed out in Chaps. 4, 5 and 6.

The relation between the individual, the community and the state is often determined by the way the past is mediated as part of public life and by the struggles that emerge in the representation of neglected social identities in practices of national remembrance. Authors like Pierre Nora (1989) and Paul Connerton (1989) have spoken about the way in which societies carry forward elements of the past, which give shape to collective memories and national identities through social commemoration and history writing. Nora has famously spoken about the *lieux de memoire*, or places of memory, which, as a result of "a play between memory and history" (1989, 19), evoke a social and political effort to remember certain aspects of the past that give meaning to a society in the present. Material or immaterial (e.g., memorials, archives, celebrations, testimonies), the preservation and signification of these sites elucidate particular visions of a collective history. In a similar manner, Connerton (1989), in his analysis of the performative aspects of social memory and its transmission, recognizes that acts of collective recollection often legitimate social orders and are driven, on many occasions, by specific political ambitions.

Following this logic, in Spain, the state's passivity towards acknowledging sites of memory from the war, the recovery of bodies, the treatment of archives, the research into the conflict, or the commemoration of the Republican defeated has demonstrated an institutional disinterest in re-signifying public versions of the history of the conflict. This has relegated the telling and writing of relevant biographies and stories to local and regional realms. Throughout the book, I engage with the question of how these forms of retelling and re-association in the exhumation archive are entwined with what Jacques Rancière (1994) terms a "poetics of knowledge." This is a practice of history that returns to the names, to specific events and to localized storytelling for the production of an all-inclusive history, that is, in effect, an intrinsically political project. As Halbwachs once described (1992), following Durkheim, their aspiration was to remember the events they had experienced and learned about socially, and to situate these histories as part of collective thought. Such shared goals, however, has not given place to a homogenous community with the same desires and aspirations. On the contrary, and as case studies have documented elsewhere, remembering violence and constructing new versions of the war-past are practices embedded in different and often intense struggles for memory (Jelin 2003).

Anthropological studies on history and memory have long argued, as David Berliner (2005, 200) points out, that people "experience and interpret their pasts from a multiplicity of viewpoints." In Spain, remembering and writing a history of defeat challenged, first of all, the dominant historical narrative around the war and postwar period perpetuated by Francoist and transitional discourses. Anthropological studies have also shown the importance of *other histories* in challenging the overbearing western notion of a single, linear, unified history (Hastrup 1992). In this regard, exhumations and the historical memory venture awakened clashing counter-narratives, to use Foucault's terms (1972), which disputed the normative and formalized versions of the Franco regime. These emerging histories created, as will be explored throughout the book, antagonisms between those who advocated the investigation of Francoist violence, and those who disputed and sometimes denied the latter's interpretation of the conflict and the violence of the dictatorship. Similarly, memories, retellings, and interpretations of the history of defeat have also been far from unanimous between historical memory associations. Appadurai (1981) and Herzfeld (1991) have emphasized how the past manifests itself as part of manifold contests over meaning in the present, and have shown how it is intricately shaped by contemporary sociopolitical milieux.

In Spain, these clashes have given place to issues of authority, continuity, antiquity, and consensus in the practice of writing and remembering the past. The interviews, commemorative events, book launches, demonstrations, and exhumation projects in which I participated revealed that such a process is fraught with political tensions at local, regional, and national levels among activist groups. In Extremadura, as elsewhere, associations often differed in terms of priorities (Ferrándiz 2006, 2011, 2013). At the core of this community was an intrinsic labour of history-making, which connected the past to the "horizon of expectations" (Koselleck 2004, 2) of a different political future. Experience and expectation, past and future, were bridged through the actions of these social collectives (ibid.), turning the construction of the past into an activity whereby democratic change could be accomplished. One of the questions with which I engaged extensively was the issue of how this novel historical production was understood, managed, and articulated. If, as Koselleck (2004) has shown, the semantics of history are entwined with the actions and ideas of the subjects and structures that produce them, then one of the main aims of this book is to examine what particular historical definitions and practices are emerging at the heart of the historical-memory venture in Extremadura. In the process of historical research into the uncertain sources of Francoist historiography, different human and non-human phenomena have become key to the social, familial, and scientific interpretation and experience of these historical events. They have also become parts of new political reformulations that challenge the status quo in local scenarios and in the context of larger national interactions.

The Ethics of Anthropological Work in Mass Grave Exhumations

Anthropology has long been concerned with issues of representation, especially in connection to ethnographic writing. Indeed, from Geertz (1975) to Clifford (1986), Rosaldo (1991), Abu-Lughod (1991), and Behar (1996), thinking about the composition of anthropological texts has meant considering the way in which the ethnographer engages with the reality of the people they study, exploring the interrelation of self and other. These debates have often dealt with ideas about the objective or subjective nature of ethnographic constructions and the power relations that determine different cultural interactions. Anthropologists such as Nancy Scheper-Hughes (1995) further consider how anthropological research and writing could be a politically engaged practice in which issues of ethics and morality become central to the work. In her famous essay for a militant anthropology, Scheper-Hughes argues that doing anthropology in the perilous situations and times in which many communities and individuals live means to carefully listen and account for these experiences with the tools of anthropology. It also means adopting an explicit "ethical orientation to 'the other'" (1995, 418) and an actively engaged position with their struggles and crises. Though some aspects of her argument have been widely criticized, I find some of Scheper-Hughes ideas around recognition in ethnographic work relevant to my own work in Extremadura.

The idea of ethnography as a practice that *recognizes* the needs of the people with whom the anthropologist collaborates has indeed informed the decisions I have made when writing this book. In the work, I have opted to use the original names of those I worked with, with their consent. Many of them, especially relatives of those killed and repressed by the Franco regime, preferred their identities to be known, as some explained, because they had already been obscured by years of public silence and institutional neglect. Most certainly, anthropological ethics committees and guidelines (see the Association of Social Anthropologists of the UK ethics guidelines for an example) often ask that anthropologists consider confidentiality in relation to the identity of collaborators, in order to protect their privacy and personal accounts. In the context of my research, issues around the exposure and visibility of information, which are key to the work of associations, scientists, and the families involved in mass grave searches, have thus been decisive when examining how best to write about people's lives and actions. In this regard, the book complies with the demands for responsibility (Scheper-Hughes 1995) that come with representing and disseminating these historical accounts and the voices of those who uttered them.

Ruth Behar (1997) and Nancy Scheper-Hughes (1995) have described ethnographic work as a way of witnessing, problematising the well-established understanding of the anthropologist as a detached observer. For Behar, for instance, notions of witnessing imply a personal connection to the observed reality, in which the "I" in ethnographic work is taken into account as it becomes entangled with the lives of the collectives and individuals it seeks to portray. The making of ethnographic knowledge, as Sheper-Hughes has highlighted, is inevitably an activity related to an act of giving testimony on the part of the observer, to an active form of eyewitnessing that places the researcher "inside human events as a responsive, reflexive and morally committed being" (1995, 419). My ethnographic contribution is thus deeply influenced by my own commitment to the study of the forms of violence and subordination that occurred in the place where I was born, to finding out about the stories of others, which, in turn, became part of my perception of my own past. Moreover, the images included in each chapter reveal a view of the exhumation intricately enmeshed with my own personal experience of each site and the relations that I formed with families, scientists, and activists alike. The choice and composition of images thus emerged not only from my conceptual preoccupations with the space of the mass grave but also from the intimate relationship I developed with it.

Through the archaeological work in the mass grave and the interviews with people who shared intensely private stories and fears with me, I too imagined and internalized these displaced forms of violence, trapped in humans, remnants, and in the landscape. My dreams and thoughts would become entangled with these fatal realities—as did those of other volunteers, neighbours, and activists—affecting my impressions and permeating my day-to-day interactions. Talking about torture, abuse, and killings in these communities provoked a particular personal response to and imagination of these forms of violence in me, which ultimately influenced the type of images I produced. In *Regarding the Pain of Others*, Susan Sontag (2003) discusses how photographs of violence have the capacity to shock audiences through the atrocities they depict and to cause particular reactions to suffering and death. Images, Sontag argues, have the power to objectify these realities but also to speak of the forms of subjectivity that generate them. Her insights into the imagery of suffering are indeed relevant in order to reflect on how one treats "the pain of others" in particular shots and compositions. The visual material in the book was difficult to produce, select, and assemble, as I was aware of the meanings that an explicit iconography of war and pain can attain in public realms, where such images, as Sontag points out, are often compulsively consumed and demanded.

Throughout each exhumation campaign, I took photographs of all the material objects, people, and moments that I considered relevant to the experience of the mass grave. I photographed familial encounters at the burials and the technical work inside the pit. Indeed, by the end of fieldwork, I had also hundreds of images of corpses, which I was not sure what to do with. At the start, I tried to avoid using pictures of bones, as whenever I showed them they seemed to attract a curiosity that had more to do with a morbid fascination around the image of the corpse and less to do with the meanings they acquired in the context of the exhumation. With time, however, and with the writing of my ethnography, I came to realize that, in the context of the chapters of the book, these images needed to be present along with those of people and of the spaces where history was invoked. The exercise of writing and "watching" (Azoulay 2008) the images I produced made me think critically about these compositions, as objects that created a space in which political engagement and negotiation was possible (ibid.). As part of a project that seeks to investigate the role of different actors in the creation of new political subjectivities and realities, I realized that my images ought also to play a role in provoking a response in the spectator.

The photographs in the book are thus another form of ethnographic representation, which allows the interpretation of violence and suffering through a different medium and language. In my attempt to work with the visual, however, I acknowledged a need to be reflective about the way in which images are used and my own position as participant and producer. It is important to recognize the value of these images in relation to the written material, since together they aim to convey the sense and meanings that corpses and stories gained in the realm of the exhumation. Likewise, ethical questions around the remaking of history after a dictatorial regime and in the current democratic milieu connect an anthropology of mass graves and exhumations with a political motivation to understand the project of families, activists, and scientists in the present. In such a way, the ethnographic work presented here is guided by an interest in examining but also engaging with these particular social realities, which are, at the same time, part of my own.

Book Outline

The chapters in the book deal with the process of exhumation as it becomes a system of information production and generate novel forms of remembrance, narrative and memorialisation. In so doing, they examine the treatment of the Republican corpse and other traces such as oral accounts and documents that are used to evidence a past that remains, still today, unrecognized.

Chapter 2 explores how the exhumations movement and the emergence of distinct human rights campaigns have engaged with historical discourses to evidence past Francoist repression and to seek the moral and symbolic recognition of victims in the present. In so doing, it considers how attempts to attain justice and state acknowledgement have been entangled with distinct judicial and institutional struggles. The chapter considers the impact that some of these contests have had on exhumation practice and on debates about the writing of history in the country.

Chapter 3 focuses, in more depth, on the present production of historical knowledge about the past in Extremadura, analysing the work of historians, archaeologists, and historical memory associations and projects in the region. The chapter deals in particular with the politics surrounding the collection of information from archives, the role of documents in historical searches, and the craft of the historian who works with the archives of the Francoist regime. Throughout this section, I establish a connection between the archive and the mass grave, connecting the work of the historian with that of the archaeologist and physical anthropologist.

Chapters 4 and 5 analyse two exhumations in the village of Castuera and Puebla de Alcocer, respectively, which are both located in the northeast of the province of Badajoz (see map of the region). The chapters examine how scientific practice, historical research, and the firsthand and inherited accounts of different generations interact to produce a history of the executions. In the case of Castuera, my analysis is concerned with the way in which collective and individual histories are produced around the unknown human remains located at the rear of the village cemetery in 2011. In relation to Puebla de Alcocer, my study is concerned with how the exhumation of the human remains of direct kin was conditioned by the persistent memory that exists about the executions and the victims in the village community.

Chapter 6 examines the way in which the enduring violence of the execution affected the lives of those related to the dead and how such violence resides at the heart of historical searches that people carry out in the present. The chapter deals with how Republican deaths haunted the lives of different generations, how they remained in the body and the mind of the living and in the artefacts and spaces connected to the war throughout the years. It considers the afterlife of repressive episodes and how they erupt in the present through the encounters that living have with the archive and the mass grave.

Chapter 7 follows the trajectory of the human remains exhumed from the mass graves to their reburial place in the municipal cemeteries of each location. The chapter explores the politics around the identification and commemoration of human remains in Extremadura, examining how the process of reburial is enmeshed with the diverse wishes of different actors and associations. It concentrates on the production of different memorials and rituals to commemorate the Civil War dead in Castuera, Puebla de Alcocer, and in a third location, Garciaz—where the search for the human remains of the missing was never accomplished. In so doing, it considers commemorative projects as sites of collective encounter but also as places of familial and political contestation.

References

Abu-Lughod, Lila. 1991. Writing Against Culture. In *Recapturing Anthropology. Working in the Present*, ed. Richard G. Fox. Santa Fe: School of American Research Press.

Aguilar Fernández, Paloma. 2008. *Políticas de la memoria y memorias de la política: el caso español en perspectiva comparada*. Madrid: Alianza Editorial.

Appadurai, and Arjun. 1981. The Past as a Scarce Resource. 16 (2): 201–219.

Assmann, Jan. 1995. Collective Memory and Cultural Identity. *New German Critique* 65: 125–133.

Azoulay, Ariella. 2008. *The Civil Contract of Photography*. New York: Zone.

Behar, Ruth. 1997. *The Vulnerable Observer: Anthropology that Breaks Your Heart*. Boston: Beacon Press.

Bell, Christine. 2009. Transitional Justice. Interdisciplinarity and the State of the "Field" or "Non-field". *International Journal of Transitional Justice* 3 (1): 5–27.

Berliner, David. 2005. The Abuses of Memory: Reflections on the Memory Boom in Anthropology. *Anthropology Quarterly* 78 (1): 197–211.

Clifford, James, and George E. Marcus. 1986. *Writing Culture: The Poetics and Politics of Ethnography*. Berkeley: University of California Press.

Coleman, Simon, and Peter Collins. 2006. *Locating the Field: Space, Place and Context in Anthropology*. Oxford: Berg.

Congram, Derek. 2016. *Missing Persons: Multidisciplinary Perspectives on the Disappeared*. Toronto: Canadian Scholars Press.

Connerton, Paul. 1989. *How Societies Remember*. Cambridge: Cambridge University Press.

Crossland, Zoë. 2013. Evidential Regimes of Forensic Archaeology. *Annual Review of Anthropology* 42: 121–137.

Crossland, Zoë, and Rosemary A. Joyce. 2015. *Disturbing Bodies. Perspectives on Forensic Anthropology*. Santa Fe: School for Advance Research Press.

Cruickshank, Julie. 1998. *The Social Life of Stories: Narrative and Knowledge in the Yukon Territory*. Vancouver: University of British Columbia Press.

Das, Veena. 2007. *Life and Words: Violence and the Descent into the Ordinary*. Berkeley, CA: University of California Press.

Derrida, Jacques. 1996. *Archive Fever: A Freudian Impression, Religion and Postmodernism*. Chicago: University of Chicago Press.

Douglas, Lee. 2014. Mass Graves gone Missing: Producing Knowledge in a World of Absence. *Culture and History Digital Journal* 3 (2): 1–12.

Dreyfus, Jean-Marc, and Elisabeth Gessat-Anstett. (eds.). 2015. *Human Remains and Mass Violence: Methodological Approaches*. Manchester: Manchester University Press.

Edwards, Elizabeth. 2014. Photographic Uncertainties: Between Evidence and Reassurance. *History and Anthropology* 25 (2): 171–188.

Encarnación, Omar G. 2008. Reconciliation After Democratization: Coping with the Past in Spain. *Political Science Quarterly* 3: 435–459.

Erll, Astrid. 2011. Locating Family in Cultural Memory Studies. *Journal of Comparative Family Studies* 42 (3): 303–318.

Etxeberría, Francisco. 2012. Prólogo. Antropología Forense de la Guerra Civil Española. *Special Issue of Boletín Galego de Medicina Legal e Forense* 18 (9): 9.

Felman, Shoshana. 2002. *The Juridical Unconscious: Trials and Traumas in the Twentieth Century*. Cambridge, MA: Harvard University Press.

Ferrándiz, Francisco. 2006. The Return of Civil War Ghosts: The Ethnography of Exhumations in Contemporary Spain. *Anthropology Today* 22 (3): 7–12.

Ferrándiz, Francisco. 2014. *El pasado bajo tierra: exhumaciones contemporáneas de la Guerra Civil*. Barcelona: Anthropos.

Ferrándiz, Francisco, and Antonius C.G.M. Robben. 2015. *Necropolitics Mass graves and Exhumations in the Age of Human Rights*. Philadelphia: University of Pennsylvania Press.

Fondebrider, Luis. 2015a. Forensic Anthropology and the Investigation of Political Violence. In *Disturbing Bodies: Perspectives on Forensic Anthropology*, ed. Zoë Crossland and Rosemary A. Joyce, 29–40. Santa Fe: School of Advance Research Press.

Fondebrider, Luis. 2015b. Forensic Anthropology and the Investigation of Political Violence: Lessons Learned from Latin America and the Balkan. In *Necropolitics. Mass Graves and Exhumations in the Age of Human Rights*, ed. Francisco Ferrándiz and Antonius C.G.M. Robben, Philadelphia: University of Pennsylvania Press.

Foucault, Michel, and Alan Sheridan. 1972. *The Archaeology of Knowledge*. London: Tavistock Publications.

Garibian, Sévane. 2015. Truth Versus Impunity: Post-transitional Justice in Argentina and the 'Human Rights Turn'. *African Yearbook of Rhetoric* 6 (1): 63–73.

Gatti, Gabriel. 2016. Lo nuestro como en *Argentina*: Humanitarian Reason and the Latin Americanization of Victimhood in Spain. *Journal of Latin American Cultural Studies* 25 (1): 147–165.

Geertz, Clifford. 1975. *Interpretation of Cultures*. London: Hutchinson.

Golob, Stephanie R. 2008. Volver: The Return of/to Transitional Justice Politics in Spain. *Journal of Spanish Cultural Studies* 9 (2): 127–141.

Halbwachs, Maurice. 1992 [1952]. *On Collective Memory*. Chicago: University of Chicago Press.

Hastrup, Kirsten. 1992. *Other Histories*. London: Routledge.

Hayner, Priscilla B. 2011. *Unspeakable Truths: Transitional Justice and the Challenge of Truth Commissions*. London: Routledge.

Herzfeld, Michael. 1991. *A Place in History: Social and Monumental Time in a Cretan Town*. Princeton, NJ: Princeton University Press.

Hirsch, Marianne. 2008. The Generation of Postmemory. *Poetics Today* 29 (1):103–128

Hirsch, Marianne. 2012. *The Generation of Postmemory: Writing and Visual Culture After the Holocaust*. New York, NY: Columbia University Press.

Jelin, Elizabeth. 2003. *State Repression and the Struggles for Memory*. London: Latin America Bureau.

Joyce, Rosemary A. 2015. Grave Responsibilities: Encountering Human Remains. In *Disturbing Bodies. Perspectives on Forensic Anthropology*, ed. Zoë Crossland and Rosemary A. Joyce. Santa Fe: School for Advance Research Press.

Juliá Diaz , Santos. 2006. Bajo el imperio de la memoria. *Revista de Occidente* (302, 303): 7–20.

Juliá Díaz, Santos. 2010. Por la autonomía de la historia. *Claves de razón práctica* 207: 8–19.

Kaplonski, Chris. 2011. Archived Relations: Repression, Rehabilitation and the Secret Life of Documents in Mongolia. *History and Anthropology* 22 (4): 431–444.

Koselleck, Reinhart. 2004. *Futures Past: on the Semantics of Historical Time*. New York: Columbia University Press.

Kovras, Iosif. 2014. *Truth Recovery and Transitional Justice: Deferring Human Rights Issues*. London: Routledge.

Kwon, Heonik. 2006. *After the Massacre: Commemoration and Consolation in Ha My and My Lai*. Berkeley, CA: University of California Press.

Lambek, Michael. 1996. The Past Imperfect: Remembering as Moral Practice. In *Tense Past: Cultural Essays in Trauma and Memory*, ed. Paul Antze and Michael Lambek. New York: Routledge.

Latour, Bruno. 1999. *Pandora's hope: Essays on the Reality of Science Studies*. Cambridge, MA: Harvard University Press.

Marcus, George. 1995. Ethnography in/of the World System the Emergence of Multi-sited Ethnography. *Annual Review of Anthropology* 24: 95–117.

Murphy, Fiona. 2011. Archives of Sorrow: An Exploration of Australia's Stolen Generations and Their Journey into the Past. *History and Anthropology* 22 (4): 481–495.

Navaro-Yashin, Yael. 2012. *The Make-believe Space: Affective Geography in a Postwar Polity*. Durham, NC: Duke University Press.

Nora, Pierre. 1989. Between History and Memory: Les Lieux de Memoire. Special Issue: Memory and Counter-Memory, *Representations* 26: 7–24.

Petrović-Šteger, Maja. 2008. Anatomising Conflict—Accommodating Human Remains. In *Social Bodies*, ed. Maryon McDonald and Helen Lambert. London: Berghahn.

Prost, Antoine. 2001. *Doce lecciones sobre la historia*. Madrid: Ediciones Cátedra.

Rancière, Jacques. 1994. *The Names of History: On the Poetics of Knowledge*. Minneapolis, MN: University of Minnesota Press.

Renshaw, Layla. 2011. *Exhuming Loss: Memory, Materiality and Mass Graves of the Spanish Civil War*. Walnut Creek: Left Coast.

Rojas-Pérez, Isaias. 2015. Unearthing Ongoing Pasts: Forensic Anthropology, State Making, and Justice Making in Postwar Peru. In *Disturbing Bodies: Perspectives on Forensic Anthropology*, ed. Zoë Crossland and Rosemary A. Joyce, 41–62. Santa Fe: School of Advanced Research Press.

Rosaldo, Renato. 1991. *Culture & Truth: The Remaking of Social Analysis*. London: Routledge.

Rosenblatt, Adam. 2015. *Digging for the Disappeared: Forensic Science After Atrocity, Stanford Studies in Human Rights*. California: Stanford University Press.

Rubin, Jonah S. 2014. Transitional Justice Against the State: Lessons from Spanish Civil Society-Led Forensic Exhumations. *The International Journal of Transitional Justice* 8 (1): 99–120.

Sanford, Victoria. 2003. *Buried Secrets: Truth and Human Rights in Guatemala*. New York, NY: Palgrave Macmillan.

Sant Cassia, Paul. *Bodies of Evidence: Burial, Memory and the Recovery of Missing Persons in Cyprus*. New York, NY: Berghahn, 2005.
Scheper-Hughes, Nancy. 1995. The Primacy of the Ethical: Propositions for a Militant Anthropology. *Current Anthropology* 36 (3): 409–440.
Sontag, Susan. 2003. *Regarding the Pain of Others*. New York: Farrar, Straus and Giroux.
Steedman, Carolyn. 2001a. Something She Called a Fever: Michelet, Derrida and Dust. *The American History Review* 106 (4): 1159–1180.
Steedman, Carolyn. 2001b. *Dust*. Manchester: Manchester University Press.
Stoler, Ann Laura. 2002. Colonial Archives and the Acts of Governance. *Archival Science* 2 (1–2): 87–109.
Stoler, Ann Laura. 2009. *Along the Archival Grain: Epistemic Anxieties and Colonial Common Sense*. Princeton, NJ: Princeton University Press.
Tarlo, Emma. 2003. *Unsettling Memories: Narratives of the Emergency in Delhi*. London: C. Hurst.
Teitel, Ruti G. 2000. *Transitional Justice*. Oxford: Oxford University Press.
Teitel, Ruti G. 2003. Transitional Justice Genealogy. *Human Rights in Transition* 16: 69–94.
Trouillot, Michel-Rolph. 1995. *Silencing the Past: Power and the Production of History*. Boston: Beacon.
Trundle, C. 2011. Searching for Culpability in the Archives: Commonwealth Nuclear test Veterans' Claims for Compensation. *History and Anthropology* 22 (4): 411–497.
Tuller, Hugh. 2015. Identification Versus Prosecution: Is it that Simple, and Where Should the Archaeologist Stand? In *Disturbing Bodies: Perspectives in Forensic Anthropology*, ed. Zoë Crossland and Rosemary A. Joyce, 85–102. Santa Fe: School for Advance Research Press.
Wagner, Sarah E. 2008. *To know Where he Lies: DNA Technology and the Search for Srebrenica's Missing*. Berkeley, CA: University of California Press.
Wouters, Nico. 2014. The Use of History in the Field of Transitional Justice: A Critical Introduction. In *Transitional Justice and Memory in Europe (1945-2013)*, ed. Nico Wouters. Cambridge: Intersentia Publishing Ltd.

CHAPTER 2

Contesting Silence, Reclaiming Historical Memory in Contemporary Spain

In 2007 several groups of families and associations submitted the cases of victims of Francoist violence to the Spanish National Court (*Audiencia Nacional*). A year later, in 2008, Judge Baltasar Garzón, who had become well-known internationally for the extradition of Augusto Pinochet in 1998, declared himself competent to investigate these complaints. Some of these cases included those of victims, which had been arrested and killed in extrajudicial executions and buried in mass graves during the Spanish Civil War (1936–1939). Others spoke of victims who had been killed in executions by firing squad resulting from death sentences in summary trials in the immediate postwar period. The complaint concluded that over 113,000 people had been killed in actions away from the battlefield—though, as many authors have argued, these crimes continued until the end of the Franco regime in 1975 (see Aguilar 2013). The judge's investigation became a landmark event because, for the first time, a Spanish court accepted cases connected to the violence perpetrated against Republicans in the period that spanned from 1936 to 1952. Moreover, the proceeding openly challenged the long-established Amnesty Law of 1977, which, during the transitional period to democracy and after Franco's death, granted freedom to left-wing political prisoners but provided full impunity to Francoist crimes (Aguilar and Ferrándiz 2016). Drawing from international human rights law, Garzón qualified these crimes as acts of enforced disappearance in the framework of crimes against humanity

Z. Aragüete-Toribio, *Producing History in Spanish Civil War Exhumations*, World Histories of Crime, Culture and Violence,
DOI 10.1007/978-3-319-61270-6_2

(Ferrándiz 2010; Closa 2013; Golob 2008; Escudero 2014), arguing that amnesty could not be applied as long as the bodies of the victims remained unfound (Closa 2013, 462).

Garzón's investigations were soon truncated. In 2009, the Director of Public Prosecutions of the National Court, accused the judge of overstepping his authority to conduct the inquiry and, in 2010, Judge Luciano Varela, from the Supreme Court, began a formal proceeding to trial the magistrate. In 2012, the Supreme Court judged Garzón on the ground of prevarication when pursuing the examination of Francoist crimes. The accusation had been promoted by the far right groups *Manos Limpias*, *Libertad y Dignidad* and *Falange Española y de la JONS*—the party that governed Spain during the Franco regime. The trial was tense, as it brought the heirs of different ideologies connected to the conflict to the same public arena. Nevertheless, it opened a new public forum where relatives of Republican victims, activists and also historians would testify to Francoist crimes for the first time since the Civil War ended in 1939. Witnesses of the defence, from second and third generations described the way in which their relatives had been detained, how they had been killed and, if they knew, the place where their bodies had been buried. In their testimonies, they coincided on the motivations to submit their complaints to the Spanish National Court: to press for an official investigation into Francoist crimes and to make these crimes known to the rest of society (*para que se sepa lo que pasó*). These collectives did not only campaign for the search for, location and exhumation of the corpses buried in known and unknown locations. They also demanded the dissemination of their stories of violence publically and the recognition of these crimes by the Spanish state and judiciary.

Since the first exhumation occurred in the year 2000—organized and led by civil society groups—a more extensive *movement for the recovery of the historical memory* has emerged, which has broken with the silence that existed in public and official milieus about past Francoist crimes. During the Franco regime, crimes committed by Republicans were investigated and trialled, with thousands of suspects sentenced to life imprisonment or death. Judicial procedures such as the *Causa General* (General Cause)—discussed later on—would compile detailed information about Republican suspects and constitute an archive to carry out the repression against the country's presumed left-wing enemy. The regime would provide Francoist victims with compensations and symbolic reparations, enabling, on many occasions, the search for, exhumation and commemoration of those who were killed by Republicans. Conversely, the mass graves of those who endured Francoist violence would remain untouched and the suffering of their families would be relegated to a private and secretive milieu. In the transitional years, as some have noted, a pact, which some have termed of silence or *pacto del olvido*, was forged between Francoist political elites and the new opposition (Aguilar 2008a), with the aim to leave the war past behind in order to attain a much awaited democratic order. This would further place the stories of Republican survivors in a marginal social space. Decisions such as the Amnesty Law of 1977; the scarce economic and symbolic reparation measures given to those who lost the war (Closa 2013; Aguilar 2008b); or the lack of an official exhumation programme to help to return human remains to Republican families rendered their experience imperceptible nationwide (Labanyi 2009).

When in 2012, Garzón was trialled, the stories of the victims of Francoist violence became the subject of strong media and political reactions worldwide, which translated Republican experiences into the language of international human rights discourses. During the trial, for example, Amnesty International stated that it was "scandalous that a magistrate was being judged for investigating human rights violations" (Lázaro 2012). The United Nations Human Rights High Commissioner, moreover, declared that "amnesty should not be provided to those responsible for crimes against humanity" (*El País* 2012). Despite the pressure exerted from international circles and the energetic backing that historical memory associations provided to Garzón nationally, in 2012, the Supreme Court dismissed the judge on the basis of a different wiretapping case for which he was also being trialled. As Rafael Escudero has observed (2014, 124), in Decision 101, in which the Supreme Court considered the authority of Judge Garzón to inquire into Francoist crimes, though the Court declared the judge not guilty of the charge of prevarication, it firmly ascertained the impossibility of inspecting "gross violations of human rights committed from 1936 to 1952" in Spain. On the one hand, the Court reminded that the Amnesty Law of 1977 was a fundamental pillar of Spanish democracy that impeded the judgement of these crimes in the present. On the other, according to Escudero (ibid.), the Court also argued that it was "legally impermissible to investigate disappearances with respect to which 'the right to know the historical truth is not part of a criminal process.'" With this statement, the Supreme Court confirmed its unwillingness to facilitate an investigation into Francoist violence, shattering the expectations of relatives and historical memory associations, and turning its back to the recommendations of international organizations.

The decision of the Supreme Court revealed the strenuous relation that the judiciary and other state institutions—as discussed later on in this chapter—have, still today, with the Civil War past and the dictatorship. In this complicated interplay, the figure of the missing, of those killed and buried in mass graves during and after the conflict, has become central to the mobilization of new legal, political, scientific and historical claims. Since the year 2000, the corpses of these left-wing Republican have been the subject of media reportages, academic study, literary writing, films, legal debates, scientific reports, political campaigns and commemorative events. Anthropologist Fráncisco Ferrándiz (2011, 532) has argued that the return of these bodies to the Spanish public realm is deeply marked by their "*radical anachronism*," as they reappeared in a society profoundly transformed by ongoing globalising and technological processes (ibid.). In Ferrándiz's words, they have erupted in a kind of "late modernity," characterized by the fast-spreading and immediate flow of information of a more complex and interconnected knowledge society. Their ubiquitous presence has thus prompted the emergence of new social meanings around their past, present and future, and pushed for the reconfiguration of politics and the law in local and national contexts.

Searching for the Recognition of Francoist Crimes

In October 2000, Madrid-based journalist Emilio Silva travelled to his father's village, Pereje, in northwest Spain, to gather information about the effects of the war in the area as part of a book he planned to write. Sixty-one years had passed since the end of the war, when Silva visited his grandmother's village with a special interest in collecting the stories of the people who, fearing death, had to flee the place and seek refuge elsewhere (other villages, other towns still under Republican rule, other countries) at the wake of Franco's military uprising. As Silva would recall later in one of his books (see Silva 2003), his own grandmother was one of the people forced to leave her house with her six children, after her husband had been executed with twelve other men in the nearby village of Priaranza del Bierzo, in 1936, in the region of Castilla y León.

The investigation into the stories of other people led Emilio to stumble upon the story of the life and death of his grandfather, Emilio Silva Faba. In *Franco's Mass Graves* (2003), Silva retells how his encounter with a friend of the family, Arsenio—a communist militant who had experienced the severe repressive reality of postwar prisons and helped him to find witnesses to the killings—marked a turning point for his search into the history of the area and into his own family's past.

After he had lunch with him one afternoon, he reminisces, "there was a moment when he told me something about the place where my grandfather's body had been abandoned and buried with twelve or thirteen other men. He also told me how they killed him and who could have been responsible for his death" (Silva 2003, 23). That day, as Silva describes, a last minute change of plans in his interview schedule led both men on the search for the mass grave where his grandfather and the other men were buried. Hours later, and after travelling around different villages and towns—to clandestine burials and cemeteries—asking elders about the existence of the mass burial, the two friends found the person who would tell them where the site was. Soon, after so many years, they would be confronted by it in person. The man pointed Silva towards a tree near the crossing of two roads. "I felt an immense emotion", writes Silva, "I walked to the tree and rested my hands on its trunk, as if in that way I could communicate with those men" (Silva 2003, 25). After locating the site, Emilio Silva and his uncle Ramón initiated the process of recovering the remains of their relative and the other corpses in the mass grave. Following an appeal to the village local authority, they received help from the town hall and soon obtained the consent of the owner of the property.

Driven by the intention to find other families who could have relatives buried in the mass grave, Emilio Silva wrote an article in the local newspaper *Crónica de León* entitled "My grandfather was also a disappeared" (*Mi abuelo también fue un desaparecido*). In it, Emilio retold the story of the detention and murder of his grandfather and expressed his intention to open up the mass grave. The article proved successful, as it allowed Emilio to find other relatives of the men in the mass grave. It also, however, raised awareness of the reality of these deaths, in a landscape of noncommittal political views around the remembrance of the war. Some authors have remarked that, throughout the decades of the 1980s and 1990s, the memory of the war, recalled publically as part of the 50th and 60th anniversaries of the conflict, was mainly imbued with the strong messages of reconciliation and consensus over the past that formed at the core of the transitional process. Gálvez Biesca (2006, 33), for instance, has called the period from 1982 to 1996, when the Spanish Socialist Workers' Party (PSOE or Socialist Pary from now on) governed the country, as the years of the "great silence" and of the "non-memory," for the question of the victims of the Civil War and the dictatorship disappeared from the party's political agenda (ibid.). In 1996, the ascent of the right-wing to the government stirred the memory of past events, making history an active tool available for political action. With the election of the conservative Popular Party (PP from now on)—some of whose members had held positions during the Franco regime—the recognition of Francoist violence became a recurrent theme in the political motions of the left-wing opposition (Humlebaek 2004).

The recovery of the human remains of Emilio's grandfather and the twelve other men buried with him in Priaranza del Bierzo made the claims for acknowledgement gain further momentum nationally and prompted an unprecedented search for the human remains of the Republican missing. Many have argued (Ferrándiz 2014, 2010; Golob 2008; Gatti 2016; Rubin 2014; Fernández Mata 2007) that this new interest in addressing the past was also entangled with broader human rights discourses and practices, which circulated transnationally at the end of the twentieth century. Among these scholars, Stephanie Golob (2008, 133) has spoken of how the development of a transitional justice consciousness worldwide, used as democratizing tool in the aftermath of conflict, also impacted on the emergence of new human rights debates in Spain. Golob (ibid.), moreover, identifies the extradition order that Judge Baltasar Garzón issued on 1998 against Augusto Pinochet, as a definitive event that "thrust Spain into the international spotlight as the very site of the globalisation of justice." The process that Judge Garzón initiated, implemented universal jurisdiction for crimes against humanity, triggering the possibility of trialling Pinochet and promoting truth-seeking in Chile. This, had also a direct effect on the collectives that began to pursue the recognition of Republican victims in Spain at the end of the 1990s, as many questioned why the Spanish judiciary had not initiated a similar procedure to investigate the human rights violations that had taken place during and after the Civil War in Spain.

In an interview with scholar Jo Labanyi (2008), Emilio explains how the Pinochet event had certainly influenced him. Reflecting back to the article he wrote in the *Crónica de León*, Emilio describes to Labanyi how his newspaper piece had aimed to show that in Spain, as in Chile, there were also "disappeared" (*desaparecidos*), for whom neither the judiciary nor the state had ever taken responsibility (Labanyi 2008b). In this way, as some have noted (Ferrándiz 2014; Rubin 2015; Gatti 2016), Emilio's article connected the Spanish Republicans killed and buried in mass graves, to the global category of victims, which emerged in relation to the crimes of enforced disappearance committed, in the '70s and '80s, in conflicts throughout the Southern Cone. More concretely, Ferrándiz (2014) and Rubin (2015) have noted how the word "disappeared" in the title of Silva's article resonated strongly with the experiences of victims in Argentina, where the term *desaparecido* referred to the abduction, confinement and disappearance of left-wing militants by the military *Junta* that ruled the country between 1976 and 1983. In this regard, Gabriel Gatti (2016) has further argued, when tracing the circulation of the term from Argentina to Spain, that the reference to the "disappeared" in Spain helped to legitimize the experiences of victims of Francoist violence, who had never been recognized as such before. In so doing, the category of "disappeared" placed those affected by Franco's violence in a global community of mourners (ibid.) and connected their suffering to that of others across post-conflict milieus.

At national level, the use of the term "disappeared" was further reinforced as more exhumations began to take place in other areas and a community around the Republican killed started to emerge. Faced with the demands of multiple families, who had also relatives buried in mass graves, Emilio created, together with Santiago Macías, a writer and activist, the *Asociación para la Recuperación de la Memoria Histórica* (Association for the Recovery of Historical Memory—ARMH from now on) in the year 2000. Two years later, in 2002, moved by the international media attention and an increasing need for logistic support, the association decided to take the case of Spain to the High Commissioner of Human Rights in the United Nations to demand the investigation of cases like Emilio's grandfather's killing by the Spanish state. After consulting with Spanish high profile human rights lawyers who had overseen claims of a same nature in Chile and Argentina, Emilio and the association compiled the cases of 75 Spanish families and a list of North American *brigadistas* who died fighting in the war—provided by the Lincoln Brigade—to present them to the UN Working Group on Enforced or Involuntary Disappearance (WGEID) at the end of that year (see also Silva 2003). As Silva recounts, the intention behind this move was to "make the problem international" (Silva 2003, 117), to increase pressure on the Spanish government and invoke their responsibility to implement an active memory politics before the United Nations. At the same time, the move exposed these cases, for the first time, to an international organization and further framed them within international definitions of enforced disappearance.

The international dimension that these cases acquired in the context of a potential UN inquiry, prompted the organization of other associations at national level, such as the *Federación Estatal de Foros por la Memoria* (Forum for Memory—Foro from now on), formed by various groups linked to the Communist Party. It also triggered the creation of regional associations and groups in places such as Extremadura or Valladolid (Labanyi 2008), and progressively all around the country. As Rubin (2015) has observed, identifying the Spanish Republican missing as "disappeared" had a powerful mobilizing effect. The entanglement of national discourses on Francoist violence with the transnational legal categories that had emerged connected to international covenants such as the Inter-American Convention on the Forced Disappearance of Persons (1994) or the 2007 International Convention for the Protection of All Persons from Enforced Disappearance (Gatti 2016) had enabled a fertile ground for action in the country. Throughout the years, international definitions of enforced disappearance were "downloaded," in the words of Francisco Ferrándiz (2010, 2014), and adapted to vernacular experiences of death and clandestine burial in Spain. These definitions were indeed decisive in the investigation that Judge Garzón launched in 2008, as they enabled the judge to argue the non-applicability of statuary limitations to these crimes, which he categorized in the framework of crimes against humanity.

Drawing on extensive historical information to document his plea, Judge Garzón argued that acts of enforced disappearance had been "systematically used [by Franco's regime] to hinder the identification of the victims and to impede judicial actions to the present day" (Ferrándiz 2010, 167). In so doing, Garzón relied on testimonies, historical analysis and archival materials that provided local meanings to the crimes Republicans had endured. His "legal reasoning" (*razonamiento jurídico*) meticulously described the legal instruments that Francoist rebels had used to justify the so-called *alzamiento nacional* or Nationalist Uprising, to depose the democratic government of the Second Republic (1931–1936) and to validate the repression against left-wing Republicans. On the one hand, the text attempted to demonstrate that "the actions carried out by those who rebelled and took part in the armed uprising of 18th July 1936, were illegal and put at risk the government" at the time, violating the principles of the constitution of 1931 (Decree 399/2006 V, 2008). On the other, the judge used historical interpretations from well-known historians and quoted key military orders to demonstrate that these killings were "consciously planned" (Closa 2013) and part of a strategy to exterminate Republican supporters. The judge referred, for instance, to the words of General Mola—who helped to plan the coup with General Franco and others—when he stated that "anyone who openly or secretly defend[ed] the Popular Front [had to] be executed" (Garzón 2008: 11, Decree 399/2006 V 2008). He also referred to the words of General Queipo de Llano—who helped advance the uprising from the south—when he said that "political leaders who escaped, would not save themselves," as he, himself, "would unearth his bodies and killed them again if they were dead" (ibid., 12).

The unsuccessful attempt of Judge Garzón to trial Francoist crimes provoked a new movement of victims' demands from national to international realms. Some of those who submitted their complaint to the Spanish National Court in 2007 referred their cases to international courts such as the European Court of Human Rights (ECHR), with the help of Spanish lawyers and legal organizations committed to the historical memory project, after Garzón was dismissed. Others groups, disappointed with the inaction of the Spanish judiciary and the equal limitations of administrative measures (further explained below), filed a complaint for the investigation of Francoist crimes, this time, in Argentina, appealing to the principle of universal jurisdiction. In 2010, the Federal Criminal and Correctional Court No. 1 in Argentina, led by Judge Maria Servini de Cubría launched the first transnational inquiry, commonly known as the Argentinian Complaint. In Spain, a new activist platform, the *Coordinadora Estatal de Apoyo a la Querella Argentina* or CeAQUA (Coordination Group in Support of the Argentinian Complaint) formed to administer the demands of relatives and associations, which submitted over 200 cases to the Argentinian Court. Vincent Druliolle (2015) has noted that one of the most significant aspects of the Complaint is that it opened the scope of the inquiry to include crimes committed between the start of the war in 1936 and the first years of the transition to democracy in 1977. This meant that the investigation would not only consider crimes of extrajudicial and judicial executions and disappearance but also, as Druliolle observes, those related to the persecution, torture, abuse and murder of left-wing activists during the second half of the Franco regime. The Argentinian Complaint would also draw on the extensive collection of testimonies from families and also survivors, some of whom would testify in Argentina in 2013 and in the Spanish National Court in 2014. The Complaint would also extract information from the *Archivo Histórico Nacional* (National History Archive) and that of the previous *Dirección General de Seguridad* (General Directorate of Security) during the Franco regime, to document, once again, human rights violations.

The Complaint, however, exposed new divisions inside the Spanish judiciary, where, though some judges have begun to collaborate, other higher judicial institutions have continued to obstruct the investigation into past Francoist violence. For instance, when Servini visited Spain in 2014, she praised the disposition of some judges in the Spanish National Court or in courts in the Basque Country and Andalucía, who had readily compiled testimonies from victims and wrongdoers. That judges were collaborating, she added "was a sign that something was profoundly changing" and that the end of impunity was soon to arrive (Torrús 2016). Nevertheless, in the last years, judges from the Supreme Court and other tribunals, have firmly opposed Servini's orders to extradite several members of the Franco regime, for instance. Moreover, in 2016, the *Fiscalía General del Estado* (Office of the Public Prosecutor) issued an extraordinary declaration that warned judges about investigating these crimes in the light of the Amnesty of Law of 1977 and reminded them of the fate of Judge Baltasar Garzón, when he initiated his own inquiry. Indeed, the adverse reaction of a great number of judges in Spain has also been the subject of critiques from international human rights actors such as Pablo De Grieff, the UN Special Rapporteur on the promotion of truth, justice, reparation and guarantees of non-recurrence, who stated his concern with the great "shortcomings" he had observed in the field of justice after visiting Spain in 2014. In his report, De Grieff (2014) reminded Spanish judges—a great number of who denied that disappearances had ever taken place in the country—of the international obligations of the country to fulfil victims' right to *justice* but also, significantly, their right to *truth*. He also urged the government and right- and left-wing parties to implement an active politics of memory that also enabled, among others, the clarification of past violent acts outside of the judicial realm.

The Politics of Historical Memory Endeavours

Since the historical memory movement began to take place at the beginning of the twenty first century, associations have demanded the reparation and recognition of Republican victims also from distinct Spanish governments. When Emilio Silva and the ARMH took the abovementioned cases to the UN Working Group on Enforced and Involuntary Disappearance (WGEID), the group requested more national institutional infrastructure to exhume and identify the corpses of the defeated; the disclosure of state files and opening of military archives; the removal of the remaining Francoist monuments; and, as Silva (2003, 189) describes in his book, the official commemoration of "all people who fought for democracy against Franco [...] so these families [could] recover their trust in politics" (Silva 2003, 189). In 2002, confronted by such appeals inside and outside of Congress, the governing leader of the conservative Popular Party (PP) at the time, José Maria Aznar, positioned his party on the issue by saying that "there was a need to leave behind the ghosts from the past, because Spaniards wanted to look to the future" (Silva 2003, 113); this is a position that the party has, to a great extent, maintained until today. Nevertheless, after much pressure from ARMH and the national and international media,[1] the Spanish Congress condemned Civil War crimes and crimes from the Franco regime on 20th of November 2002—a symbolic date that at once commemorated the deaths of the dictator General Francisco Franco and the death of the founder of *Falange Española*, José Antonio Primo de Rivera. As Silva recalls in his book, this was an important step towards the moral recognition of the families that suffered not only the loss and death of relatives but also all those whose lives were affected by the dictatorship's violent rule (i.e., life-sentenced prisoners, forced-labour workers, exiles, or abused women, to cite but a few examples).

Over the years, the demands expressed to the UN working group formed the common objectives for the historical memory movement, which strengthened the aim of creating a new social reality for those affected by the history of defeat in the country. As Sergio Gálvez Biesca (2006, 36) has pointed out, these common objectives were consolidated over time to include (1) the moral, judicial and economic reparation of the victims by national institutions; (2) the nullity of all Francoist judicial procedures; (3) a final solution to the exhumation of mass graves; (4) the eradication of "the Francoist nomenclature and symbolism" in villages and towns and (5) the creation of an archive of the Civil War and the dictatorship. After much campaigning, many of these initial demands for restoration on the part of associations such as ARMH, the Foro, and other regional and family groups finally obtained a response when the Socialist Party was re-elected in 2004. Stephanie Golob (2008) and Paloma Aguilar (2008b), for instance, have noted that during the socialist mandate from 2004 to 2008, Spain witnessed the first initiatives that dealt with the suffering of Republican victims in the form of "post-transitional justice" mechanisms. Moreover, these authors also explain how such initiatives developed in connection to particular interests inside the party to reform the democratic status quo. Golob (2008, 133) observes that restorative measures were created as part of a political programme that intended to redefine Spanish citizenship by "expanding rights for groups either historically ignored or treated unequally by the central government." Moreover, Aguilar (2008b) has further argued that some of the symbolic reparations that PSOE envisioned were proposed not only by the group but also by its president, José Luis Rodriguez Zapatero, whose grandfather was a Republican officer killed by Francoist supporters (ibid.; Golob 2008).

In 2004, when PSOE was elected, an Interministerial Commission was created to "repair and restore the dignity and memory of the victims of the Civil War and the dictatorship" (Macé 2012, 765). According to the government's online platform on historical memory,[2] the goal of the commission was to study their situation, in order to create a new law, to provide different forms of economic and symbolic reparations and to enable the access to archives. In a climate of divergent political positions in relation to the war past, the parliamentary debates surrounding the draft law were tense and convoluted. Analysing news items from this time, Jean François Macé (2012) has noted how the first recommendations of the Commission were soon strongly critiqued by the conservative Popular Party, who accused Rodriguez Zapatero of seeking revenge and aiming to divide Spanish people. The possibility that these crimes might be officially acknowledged and symbolically atoned shook the Spanish right-wing and its organizations profoundly. Macé (ibid.) has further explained how, around this period, representatives of some of the most traditional Francoist groups openly manifested their will to continue venerating the figure of the dictator and remained loyal to the memory of Francoism.[3] In view of these opposing positions, Rodriguez Zapatero reminded the country publically, in 2005, that Republican victims should be acknowledged for they had suffered the effects of a military regime, in silence, over 40 years. Nevertheless, the work of the Commission also provoked the discontent of left-wing groups such as *Izquierda Unida* (United Left, IU) or *Esquerra Republicana de Catalunya* (Republican Left of Catalonia, ERC), which critiqued the legal project for its lack of ambition (ibid.).

In an effort to reassert the commitment of the executive to the recognition of the Republican past, the government of Rodriguez Zapatero declared 2006 the year of "historical memory." Moreover, the same year, the Permanent Commission of the Parliamentary Assembly of the Council of Europe unanimously condemned the Franco regime and demanded that its victims were recognized by the government and the country's political elites (Aguilar 2008b; Escudero 2014). Amnesty International would also exert pressure on the Spanish government through several reports in 2005, 2006a and 2006b (Aguilar 2008b), which denounced the lack of aid to Republican victims, the concerns of the organization with regards to the draft law and the situation of state archives, respectively. In 2007, a year after Spain signed the UN International Convention for the Protection of all Persons from Enforced Disappearance, the Spanish parliament finally passed the Law 52/2007, technically known as the "*Law of 26th of December through which the rights and measures in favour of those who suffered persecution or violence during the civil war and dictatorship are recognised*," with the abstention of PP and ERC. The new measure legislated and provided funding for the exhumation of mass graves and the identification of human remains; regulated the heritage and memorialisation of the conflict in the country, addressing the issue of Francoist monuments[4] and the future of the Valley of the Fallen, the funerary complex where Franco and over 34,000 corpses from both sides of the conflict remain buried today; amplified the economic compensation given to victims during the transition to democracy; and issued official moral recognition declarations to those who endured the violence of the war and the Franco regime.

Once it was put into force, the much-awaited law met with the objections and disappointment on the part of many associations (Ferrándiz 2013) and some human rights organizations. As the response of the director of Amnesty International in 2007, Esteban Beltrán stated, "the law constituted a timid move forward in the long fight against the forgetting of victims of Francoism and the Civil War" and added that, "without truth and justice the debt will never be settled" (Amnesty International 2007). Most analysts (see Chinchón 2012: 36; Martin Pallín 2011; Escudero 2011) have also agreed that the law falls short in relation to the moral reparation and rights of families and survivors, as it does not consider Franco's repression from a judicial perspective. The law, for instance, does not deal with issues of accountability and the court investigation of the crimes committed. In fact, the legal text asserts that the law does not seek to sanction the crime of enforced disappearance but instead to promote knowledge of the past "within the framework of the spirit of reconciliation" (Law 52/2007, 96, cited in Ferrándiz 2010). In addition to this, the act did not annul Francoist sentences, as historical memory collectives had demanded, and instead declared them "unjust" and illegitimate (Macé 2012, 770; Ferrándiz 2014). In this context, many of these groups felt, as Francisco Ferrándiz has argued, that the measure never fully complied with their requests for "truth, justice, and reparation" and the "dismantling of the 'Spanish impunity system'" (Ferrándiz 2013, 45).

Moreover, with regards to truth-seeking practices such as exhumations, for instance, the state would provide only limited administrative assistance and funding for the location and excavation of mass graves, addressing vaguely aspects about the unearthing and treatment of human remains. In essence, the law established what Francisco Ferrándiz (2013, 45) has termed as a "human rights outsourcing system" that made associations and family groups responsible for the organization of archaeological interventions and the ensuing identification of corpses. Indeed, the law 55/2007, most commonly known as Law of Historical Memory, facilitated the funding of multiple exhumation and identification projects but also activities connected to the compilation of historical material, the elaboration of a census of victims, the dissemination of historical studies through publications, the production of films and the organization of conferences, seminars and exhibitions (Ministry of Justice 2007). Nevertheless, it derived all responsibility for these endeavours to families, local associations and to some of the institutional projects that had been created regionally since the exhumation movement had begun in the year 2000. Throughout the years, institutional projects of different nature had emerged in places such as Extremadura, Andalusia, the Basque Country, Catalonia or Galicia, in which families' demands for the location and exhumation of missing relatives and historical research about the killings were dealt with by regional administrations, with the support of experts and academics (Ferrándiz 2014, 81). This, of course, was not the case in all regions. Instead, one could say that the lack of a consistent response from the central state has created an uneven landscape of practices, research infrastructure and exhumation resources in the last two decades.

In 2011, with the return of the Popular Party (PP) to the government, the provisions made by the Law of Historical Memory, including the grants for exhumations, were gradually dismantled. In 2012, the new government cut the funding for historical memory initiatives from 6.5 million to 2.5 million euros per year. In the new budget, as the government of the Popular Party argued, the funds would be entirely dedicated to the exhumation of mass graves, eliminating the sum of money provided for other historical research and dissemination activities. Considering that the socialist government of Rodriguez Zapatero had destined 1.3 million to the development of exhumations, PP presented the new budgetary adjustment as a positive change, as more money would be accordingly dedicated to the location of victims in mass graves. Nevertheless, that year, no calls for exhumation projects were issued in the *Boletín Oficial del Estado* (Official Bulletin of the State), leaving family groups and historical memory associations without resources for the excavation of war and postwar mass burials (Junquera 2013). Moreover, in 2012 the PP government also closed the Victims' Office that the Socialist Party had opened to deal with the demands and queries of families and survivors in 2008. In 2013, PP Minister of Justice, Alberto Ruiz-Gallardón, explained to the press that funding had been cancelled due to budgetary restraints—in the light of the economic crisis and ensuing recession that the country had experienced since 2008. The minister also stated that support had been eliminated because most major exhumations had already been carried out during the Socialist Party's term in office (Junquera 2013).

Once again, between the years of 2013 and 2016, the government assigned no budgetary allocations for Civil War exhumations. This led families and associations to rely on alternative sources of funding such as crowdfunding bids or donations from private and international benefactors. In his report, issued in 2014, the UN Special Rapporteur Pablo De Grieff lamented the government's inaction towards the demands of victims, which historical memory associations continued to receive. Indeed, the lack of funding and support impacted on the timings and procedures of historical memory projects. State inaction triggered the participation of more families in the Argentinian Complaint (Ryan 2016). It also generated the drafting of new laws at regional level that aimed to secure the appropriate continuation of exhumations and to safeguard rights and reparation of those who endured Francoist violence. In 2013, for instance, the region of Navarra approved the Foral Law of Historical Memory, which, according to Lorraine Ryan (2016, 6), aimed to compensate for the "deficiencies" of the national law, covering the cost of exhumations, providing technical support and enabling the reburial of the corpses. Around the same time, a similar initiative was proposed in the region of Andalusia, where a new Law of Historical and Democratic Memory would be negotiated in parliament. In this case, the draft law established that the *Junta de Andalucía* (Government of Andalusia) would promote exhumations and also sanction any attempts to destroy mass graves or contravene exhumation projects. In both instances, both regional draft laws contemplated the cultural management of conflict heritage and proposed the formation of a DNA bank for the identification of missing victims.

The study of exhumations presented here focuses on a period during which governmental funding was still available. Many of the excavations I followed in Extremadura were indeed financed through the grants provided to local family groups and historical memory associations by the national government of the Socialist Party between 2009 and 2011. Nevertheless, the case of Extremadura is also relevant because, as explored in the following chapters, civil society collectives counted with the aid of an institutional project, which provided help with the search for, exhumation and identification of human remains and the historical investigation of these repressive acts. In Extremadura, one could also observe the micro-politics at play in the process of exhumation, as institutional agendas, party programmes and the goals and wishes of relatives and historical memory associations needed to be negotiated during each excavation project. Most certainly, as the next chapters show, the exhumation of mass graves and the memorialisation of the Civil War are contested terrains in which manifold actors promote divergent—though not incommensurable views—of what it means to recover the bodies of the Republican killed, today. A close look at the social dynamics of the exhumation process reveals how these corpses and their historical signification are entangled with different political aspirations that encompass those of individual actors, political groups and state agents. At the core of the exhumation project, one can observe how such political claims confer, interact and, on occasions, collide with one another as well as with the scientific expertise that has led excavations since the year 2000.

Exhuming the Human Remains of the Republican Defeated

Generally, institutional and civil society initiatives have drawn from the experience of other post-conflict contexts to develop vernacular practices around the exhumation of human remains or the preservation and memorialisation of war and postwar heritage in Spain (Ferrándiz 2011, 2013, 2014; González Ruibal 2007, 2009; Viejo Rose 2011). Francisco Ferrándiz (2013, 2014, 17) has observed, for instance, that with regards to exhumations, scientific teams in Spain have used international guidelines on exhumation of human remains, following the method of operation of other established forensic groups such as the Argentinean Forensic Anthropology Team (EAAF) and others. From the start of the twenty first century, exhumation work has been guided, according to Francisco Etxeberría (2003), one of the leading forensic experts in Spain, by covenants such as the 1991 United Nations Manual for the Prevention and Investigation of Extra-legal, Arbitrary and Summary Executions; the previous 1989 United Nations Principles for the Investigation of Extrajudicial, Arbitrary and Summary Executions; or the 1992 Declaration for the Protection of All Persons against Enforced Disappearances, among others. Speaking of memorialisation practices in Spain, González Ruibal (2009) has noted how forms of re-interpreting the cultural heritage of the conflict and the dictatorship can vastly draw from similar examples in post-Holocaust Germany or South Africa. Along the same lines, Viejo Rose (2011) has compared processes of social reconstruction in post-war and post-Franco Spain to those in countries like Bosnia, observing how the re-signification of previous forms of heritage is a varied exercise that contributes to the rewriting of dominant historical versions of past events.[5]

Nevertheless, in the vernacular processes of remembrance and of re-definition of the past that take place in Spain, conflicting views and disagreements have also emerged, at local level, among family groups and historical memory associations. In the early days of the exhumation movement and with the initial media fuzz (Ferrándiz and Baer 2008), issues around how best to interpret, record and remember the war past came to the forefront of disputes between members of grassroots collectives in Spain. On the one hand, images of the first archaeological interventions, which exposed corpses and the visible traces of violence on their bones, prompted a negative attitude towards the unearthing of human remains. As some authors have pointed out (Ferrándiz 2014: 61) associations such as the Association of the War Archive and Exile (AGE) opposed the practice of unearthing the remains because it considered that exhuming these mass graves was like "erasing genocide" (ibid.). Likewise, other collective and individual voices defended a non-interventionist approach to the mass graves of the conflict, arguing instead for the memorialisation of such sites with monoliths or other markers. This proposed alternative treatment of the unmarked burial sites understood the inscription of these places as a way of making mass graves visible around the Spanish territory. For some, these markers acted as evidence (Ferrándiz 2007; Fernández de Mata 2011) of the executions committed by the Francoist rearguard—as one interviewee explained to me at the beginning of my fieldwork. Similarly, vestiges such as street names, monuments or the infamous Valley of the Fallen have also been the focus of strong controversies: Some have challenged their place in present-day Spain, others have demanded their re-signification, and revisionist voices have advocated their historical and sentimental value for the country (Aguilar 2008a; Macé 2012; González Ruibal 2009; Ferrándiz 2014).

As time went on, discrepancies also emerged between members of the pro-exhumation movement, especially with regards to the appropriate procedures and actions to follow "*below ground*" (Ferrándiz 2006, 2010, 2013, 2014), in relation to the exhumation and reburial of human remains. This is apparent, for instance, in the different views that the two main national associations, namely ARMH and the Foro, entertain of the exhumation process. For ARMH the reasons for the excavation and reburial of human remains have mainly been connected to the need for families to recover the corpses of their ancestors. In its approach, the association emphasizes the kinship bond of children and grandchildren with their disappeared relatives over the political affiliation of the dead, promoting the idea that exhumations have the potential to heal and offer closure on traumatic pasts (Bevernage and Colaert 2014). Conversely, the Foro aims to help families recover the human remains of their *militant* relatives, reclaiming, first and foremost, their political identities. This follows the founding ethos of the association, which, connected to the Communist Party, was born "clearly linked to the left-wing […] with a strong conviction to fight against the forgetting of the defeated"—as stated on the website of the association. According to Bevernage and Colaert (2014, 6), who examine the divergent understandings of the exhumation process between both associations, the Foro does not place the same emphasis on the reparation of collective trauma. Instead, they have what the authors acknowledge as a clear interest in the teaching of a political history through exhumations, with the hope that political realities like that of the Second Republic might regenerate in the future.[6]

Francisco Ferrándiz (2010, 2013, 2014) has observed that these disparities ultimately manifest in the "political and mortuary rituals" (Ferrándiz 2006) that each group employs in the location of burials, their excavation and in the reburial of corpses. As Ferrándiz notes, for ARMH, relatives "are autochthonous and definitive in the organization of mourning" (ibid., 9). In the exhumations and reburials of the Foro the politicization of these acts prevails and is apparent through the left-wing symbolism used, such as flags, songs and hymns, or the political speeches uttered (ibid.). To these contrarieties, one has to add particular wishes for other types of remembrance and commemoration (e.g., religious) that might clash with the agenda of some associations. Such social and political differences have also, ultimately, conditioned and been conditioned by the scientific work and the other forms of historical knowledge production performed in connection to the mass grave. On many occasions, scientific practice has emerged as a tool for claiming authority between competing associations. For instance, according to Ferrándiz (ibid.), associations like ARMH and the Foro increasingly expanded their links with experts in the fields of forensic anthropology, archaeology and other social sciences in an effort to "defend themselves against reciprocal accusations of non-professional conduct and to give their exhumations a more 'scientific' and thus legitimate character" (Ferrándiz 2006, 9; see also González Ruibal et al. 2015). On the other hand, scientific and other activities such as historical research into archives, publications, presentations, or exhibitions have also served to disseminate information about the repression that the mass graves point towards, in order to contravene recent revisionist voices.

ARMH, the Foro, and their local and regional branches around the country have promoted most of the searches for the human remains of the missing, their reburial and appropriate tributes. In so doing, they have worked with different, often, interdisciplinary scientific groups comprised of archaeologists, physical and forensic anthropologists, biologists, historians and social anthropologists. Such is the case of the forensic team of the *Sociedad de Ciencias Aranzadi*, led by forensic scientist Francisco Etxeberría and funded by the government of the Basque Country; the group led by biologist Luis Ríos at the Complutense University in Madrid; or the team managed by archaeologist Réne Pacheco, as part of ARMH. Other examples include the team supervised by archaeologist Juan Montero Caminero in Burgos University; the team of Laura Muñoz Encinar, who was in charge of exhumations in Extremadura between 2005 and 2014; or the team of Alfredo González Ruibal in the *Instituto de Ciencias del Patrimonio* (Institute of Heritage Science or INCIPIT). All these teams, as Francisco Ferrándiz (2014) has pointed out, have also developed, throughout the years, specific methodologies that comply with international protocols and which address the needs proper to the Spanish context. The inconsistent memory politics of distinct left- and right-wing governments generated a lack of a unified approach to regulating the scientific activity in mass graves.

Over the years, the lack of an official scientific committee to endorse expert work in exhumations has also generated other problems for archaeological and forensic teams. González Ruibal et al. (2015) have pointed out, more recently, that this lack of support on the part of the state has complicated the work of archaeologists and other scientists, as the absence of regulation, makes some question the need for professionals to carry out excavation and exhumation work. Most certainly, the release of a national protocol in 2011—before the end of the Socialist mandate—meant the instauration of a general set of guidelines to be used in regions where local protocols had not yet been created. Such protocol also drew from the previous 1991 UN procedures but was, in the eyes of many, an insufficient measure, which came too late and years after well-developed methodologies had already been put in place by the most active teams. On the ground, however, as González Ruibal et al. (2015) explain, this has given place to tensions between those who demand excavation projects; those who, being trained as archaeologists, work in excavations for free; and professional teams that are paid to carry out these tasks. These collectives, as the authors observe, often clash in relation to the symbolic and economic value of the archaeologist's work, as those professionals who work on a voluntary basis look at paid archaeologists with suspicion, and other members of historical memory associations sometimes consider the cost of archaeological expertise too high (ibid., 123). In this situation, the authors have feared that the isolation of these practices by the central government and the disapproval of expert work in some local circles might lead to weakening "the impact of archaeology [and related scientific practices], hinder[ing] the dissemination of results, lower[ing] professional standards, and foster[ing] socio-political atomization" (ibid., 124).

Scientists have vindicated the need for expert knowledge and know-how in exhumations since the beginning of the exhumation campaign. In the year 2000, two of the exhumation experts that collaborated with Emilio Silva in the search for and excavation of the human remains of the thirteen men buried in Priaranza del Bierzo, archaeologist Julio M. Vidal Encinas and anthropologist Maria Encina Prada Marchos, published an article in which they expressed some early remarks about the aims and methods to be followed in relation to Civil War exhumations. In "An Archaeology of Reconciliation", the two scientists express their commitment to exhumations in order to "comply with the yearnings of those who want to recover the bodies of their relatives" (2002, 1). In it, the authors further emphasize the importance of a painstaking methodology to secure, as they see it, a "professional" treatment of the mass grave and to avoid improper procedures that might destroy these interments. Scientists in general have been constant in their efforts to collect, organize and preserve evidence of these executions. In following years, Francisco Etxeberría has often reinforced this point in public presentations and in publications (2003, 2005). For the forensic doctor, the adherence to professional practice is paramount in order to produce adequate evidence of the acts of violence that took place during and after the war. He has written that disciplines such as anthropology and paleopathology should aim to "produce the maximum information for the clarification of truth" with a view to contributing to any possible future judicial process or a truth commission in the country (2005, 538).

The specific focus on the appropriate production of evidence has engaged scientists with a clear forensic approach to the exhumation of mass graves—even if exhumations do not take place in the context of a judicial investigation. Scientific objectives of exhumation work have remained circumscribed to attaining the ultimate official recognition of past crimes. As Adam Rosenblatt (2015) has observed, recently, contexts where human rights violations have taken place have transformed the nature of forensic work worldwide, as, on many occasions, such practices have occurred in the margins of official action and in precarious situations. In other scenarios, they have ultimately triggered processes of judicial inquiry in their aftermath (i.e., Argentina or Guatemala). Due to the decentralized approach to exhumations, in Spain, scientists have further warned of the need to appropriately collect historical information in archives and through testimonies and to follow informed approaches to the archaeological intervention in mass graves and the anthropological study of human remains. Moreover, some have reminded to the need to write and store results in a thorough manner, in order to furnish future, yet uncertain, institutional processes (Etxeberría 2003; Leizaola 2006). Etxeberría (Leizaola 2006) has remarked, the significance of these two aspects, because "anything that is not written is as if it did not exist" (ibid.) and because new repositories should be created to accommodate the different analyses that emerge from the mass grave (ibid.). In a similar manner, Alfredo González-Ruibal (2009, 108) has spoken about the need to historicise the information that is being produced in the mass grave, to publicize the results and to make "a coordinated effort to provide Spain with a spatial and material memory culture." In this view, the exhumation is a key place for remembrance but also for the production of "History, in capital case" (ibid., 110). A space that, in the view of the archaeologist, should be treated through a "total archaeological approach [...] that delves into the past, favours the preservation of its material footprints and contributes to disseminating history in a critical and comprehensive way" (ibid.). The argument of Francisco Etxeberría and Alfredo González Ruibal resonates with the approach that I encountered in Extremadura during fieldwork, where the information extracted from mass graves was treated as potential evidence for a judicial process but also for the historical investigation that the project with which I collaborated developed.

Both views of the exhumation process are illustrative of the importance that mass graves attained in the creation of knowledge about the Civil War and postwar past. These arguments also indicate a concern for the production of truth, even beyond the exhumation of mass graves. The unearthing of the human remains of the defeated has also been surrounded by the intense publication of academic but also non-academic works, many of which have been made available under the rubric of historical memory. Many have challenged the idea that some of these productions bring new information about the events that took place during the conflict. Some, as explained later on, have criticized them for their lack of rigour and, on occasions, for their sentimentalism (Aróstegui 2009; Fernández de Mata 2007; Juliá 1999, 2006), advocating the professional approach of the historian to carry out the research and writing of history. For others involved in the historical memory movement, exhumations and the knowledge production process that developed around them gave place to what some people I met during fieldwork saw as a democratization of the practice of history. Many felt that access to this past had been enabled through the historical memory venture, making the exercise of history not only the task of professional scholars but also of non-university based historians and amateurs. The exhumation awakened the need for many to partake in the construction of new meanings about the past, especially as such troubled history was part of localized political, personal and social life histories. As González Ruibal et al. (2015, 133) have remarked, in this context, exhumations processes have unveiled wider social tensions in relation to who has the "right to produce knowledge" about past events and "under what circumstances." They have enabled a public space in which narratives can be articulated, contested and re-shaped by the multiple voices that have begun to take part in the research of the Spanish contemporary past.

Historical Memory and the Research of the Civil War Past

Producing historical narratives about the forms of violence that left-wing Republicans endured has become a central tenet for those involved in exhumations and other forms of memorialisation because, for many years, the history of the conflict remained entangled with the dominant version of the past imposed by the Franco regime. For some historians (Preston 1999; Chaves Palacios 2000; Blanco Rodriguez 2007), historical production during the dictatorship was clearly relegated to serve the propagandistic aims of the fascist government. Others scholars such as Gil Vico (1998) have further highlighted how this propagandistic will was bolstered by judicial processes that were used to collect information on left-wing suspects after the conflict. For instance, processes such as the so-called *Causa General* (General Cause)—established by decree on 26th April 1940—aimed to amass details about the crimes committed by Republican left-wing militants and supporters and their political affiliation (Gil Vico 1998). In so doing, the investigation built an important registry that would later be used to carry out the persecution and repression of left-wing Republicans and to nurture the trials of Military Tribunals (see Chaves Rodriguez 2015; Aguilar 2013). Such an archive of personal, professional and political information about Republicans also constituted a fundamental technology of ideological persuasion which reminded Spanish people of the obligation to manifest an "open connection with the regime" (Gil Vico 1998, 179).[7] The *Causa General* and other military (Chaves Rodriguez 2015) and ordinary trials (Aguilar 2013) provided accounts that delineated the contours of a Republican enemy, which the regime yearned to contain and eliminate. Gil Vico (1998, 179) remarks that the procedure helped the new state to create a narrative of domination, which extended a view of the Second Republic as a "loathsome regime of murderers" inside and outside of Spain.

Out of this process came publications of a historical character such as *La Dominación Roja en España* (Red Domination in Spain), published in 1943, and *Datos Complementarios para la Historia de España: Guerra de Liberación (1936–1939)* (Complementary Information for the History of Spain: Liberation War (1936–1939)), published in 1945 in Spain and a year later, for English and Latin American audiences. Both of these books, according to Gil Vico (1998, 183), sought to prove that the uprising was "providential," reinforcing the narrative of liberation that Francoist followers had promoted during the war. According to Paul Preston (1999, 164), in the most immediate years after the struggle, the Francoist establishment elaborated a narrative that portrayed the war as a religious "crusade" (*cruzada*) that had restored a Catholic moral and hierarchical order against what they considered a Republican anarchic and atheist society. The message of the regime, as many have argued (Fernández de Mata 2007; Richards 2011; Preston 2011; Ferrándiz 2014), vindicated the salvation of Spain from the foreign Bolshevist, Masonic, and Jewish influence (Preston 2011; Richards 2011) that presumably operated in the country during the Second Republic (1931–1936). Moreover, it professed that the fundamental pillars of the nation, namely "Religion, Fatherland, Family, and Property" had been reinstated (Preston 1994, 41; Juliá 1979) after the war had ended. In this interpretation of the conflict, Republican families and survivors became known and classified as the anti-Spain and also as *reds*, (Fernández de Mata 2007: 202)—categories that rendered these groups second-class citizens in Spain's postwar society. With time, Republican victims and survivors would feel, in the words of Ignacio Fernández de Mata (2007, 203), as the "Civil War forgotten".

Historical works were, for many years, relegated to the writings of historians connected to the Franco regime. This created a difficult situation for the research and writing of a comprehensive history of the Second Republic, the Civil War and the dictatorship (Preston 1999; Juliá Díaz 2006). Santos Juliá (2006) has spoken of the lack of disposition to investigating this period and, especially, the history of defeat, in the 1950s, as many national historians avoided stepping into the ground of twentieth century events. During the '60s and '70s, strong censorship consigned historical production to overseas academics (historians and Hispanists such as Hugh Thomas, H.R. Southworth or Gabriel Jackson, to name a few) who offered innovative accounts though with a tendency to generalize about the conflict (Blanco Rodriguez 2007). Authors such as Paul Preston (1999), Julián Chaves Palacios (2000) or Juan Andrés Blanco Rodriguez (2007) have noted that foreign researchers counted with invaluable media sources abroad as well as the testimonies of those that had exiled after the war, which enabled them to carry out their research. Nevertheless, at this time, national and local archives remained still extremely difficult to access. As these authors explain, only those who sympathized with the regime could use them for their state-sponsored research. Santos Juliá (2006) has reflected that for the generation of Spanish historians who grew up during the dictatorship and would later write more nuanced accounts of the conflict and the regime, Francoist versions of the Civil War soon became known as representations of the past based on "lies" and on the particular memory that "others" had imposed from above.

Historical studies by national researchers about the period of the Second Republic and the Civil War began to emerge, especially, after the death of the dictator (Juliá Díaz 2006). This new current of researchers pushed for the development of historical production towards more detailed inquiries of social, political and economic character. During the '80s and '90s, numerous publications appeared coinciding with the fiftieth and sixtieth anniversary of the beginning and end of the war; some information repositories in governmental institutions as well as in national, regional and municipal archives[8] (Blanco Rodriguez 2007) were opened to researchers; and new testimonies emerged. In 1999, historian Santos Juliá edited the book *Víctimas de la Guerra Civil* (Victims of the Civil War), which offered one of the first nuanced accounts of the deaths resulting from clandestine and extrajudicial killings perpetrated by Francoist forces during the Civil War (Chaves Palacios 2000). Other local studies at the time also contributed to creating new knowledge about the names and numbers of Republican victims that were killed in *sacas* or *paseos* (ibid.). Years later and after exhumations began in the 2000s, other important regional works emerged—some of which included exhaustive lists with information about those who had been killed in extrajudicial and judicial executions. In southern Spain, for instance, one of the most well-known publications of the kind was *La Columna de la Muerte* (The Column of Death) published by historian

Francisco Espinosa Maestre in 2003. Espinosa's work constitutes a meticulous study, village by village, of the advance of the Francoist army through Andalusia and Extremadura, and provides a detailed account of the killings that occurred in these localities.

Though the *Causa General* constituted a thorough inquiry that enabled the recording of the deaths of Francoist victims on civil registries, no state count exists to this date of the number of Republican victims killed in extrajudicial executions. This was one of the points raised by the UN Special Rapporteur, Pablo De Grieff, in the report he produced in 2014, which regretted the lack of "official censuses of victims, or data or official estimates of the total number of victims of the Civil War and the dictatorship" (2014, 10). The historiography of the regime had made constant efforts to address the question of casualties during the conflict but these numbers were often dissonant and imbalanced, and again, subject to the regime's agenda and doctrine. For instance, some of the most notable works realized by Franco's biographer and historian Ricardo de la Cierva, estimated that, during the Civil War, 100,000 victims had perished in both flanks and that 50,000 victims had been killed as a result of forms of extrajudicial repression. Of this number, according to the author, 8000 people would have been killed as a result of Francoist violence (Reig Tapia 1984, 80). Presumably, as some scholars have remarked later on (see Reig Tapia 1984), these figures had been "borrowed" from the inquiries of another historian of the regime, Ramón Salas Larrazábal, whose most renowned work, *Pérdidas de la Guerra Civil* (Civil War Casualties), published in 1977, offered the most systematic count of victims in both flanks until that date. The results of this work, as Chaves Palacios (2000) has noted, would soon be challenged later on by other studies in particular areas such as La Rioja, Almería or Extremadura.

In recent years, the work of historians has become especially relevant in historical memory campaigns. Works such as Espinosa Maestre's have become widely read by families, activists and Civil War enthusiasts and referenced by other historians and academics. Blanco Rodriguez (2007, 25) remarked that with the search for the Republican missing the history of the conflict gained "an important social presence." Historical work shed new light over these killings, and most importantly, over the information held in civil registries, military archives and other sources. It also drew from multiple testimonies that began to emerge offering new accounts about irregular and institutionalized forms of repression, the experience of prisons and concentration Camps, or stories from the war front. In the last two decades, families and historical memory activists have often engaged in a dialogue with historians in order to locate information about a person's life, death or disappearance. Likewise, archaeologists, physical anthropologists and forensic experts have also relied on the research of historians to analyse the context of the mass grave and the executions from which these mass burials resulted. Historical research also became central in the unsuccessful judicial processes that have taken place in the country. Some historians, for instance, participated in the trial of Baltasar Garzón and in the investigation of Argentinian Judge Maria Servini de Cubría. These legal processes have contributed, as some have noted of similar contexts elsewhere, to the judicializaton of history in the context of trials for human rights violations. Historical analysis has thus acquired an active role in the quest for the recognition of these episodes and for the redress of those who suffered them.

Nevertheless, within the field of history, different debates have surfaced, in the last years, about the relationship that the discipline should have with the historical memory phenomenon. Indeed, some have challenged both the notion of "historical memory" and the involvement of historians in these campaigns. The emergence of new voices from generations which experienced the conflict indirectly or who feel a strong commitment to disseminating stories about the Francoist repression has given place to new written productions and historical works published under the rubric of "historical memory." Historians such as Santos Juliá (2006, 2010), for instance, have critiqued the use of this term widely, alleging that what has often been referred to, in recent years, as historical memory does not refer to memory but in fact history. Some have argued (see Colom González 2010) that, for Juliá, historical memory implies an epistemological confusion between "remembering" and "knowing." Santos Juliá (2006, 2010) understands memory as that which is confined to the realm of the individual and to a personal experience of past events. Influenced by historiographic debates on the uses of memory in twentieth century France (e.g., Nora (1989), Todorov ([1995] 2000), the author associates historical memory—which he understands as a form of collective memory—to public discourses and practices of remembrance tainted by the desires and politics of those who promote them. Contrary to this idea, Juliá presents history as the only possible vehicle to know the past objectively and rigorously. In his approach to history, he also reclaims the significance of the historical method and the ability of the professional historian, as the author (2010, 17) explains citing Marc Bloch, to retell how "things really happened".

Other scholars such as Francisco Colom González (2010) have critiqued Juliá's understanding of historical memory arguing that, though the term can indeed be problematic, Juliá undermines the value that it has gained for Spanish contemporary society. For Colom González historical memory has more to do with a debate around the "moral and political significance of collective remembrance" than with historical accuracy. Through the historical memory campaign, the author explains, Spanish people have aimed to face a past of traumatic events and to reconcile with it. In this respect, such concept is intimately connected to a desire for collective reparation, which is entangled with the political aspirations of some but also with a societal demand, on the part of those affected by Francoist repression, to have their experiences acknowledged publically. Historical work has become, in this context, an important means of expression and also, a source of knowledge in order to confront Francoist claims about past crimes. Such role has also been criticized by Santos Juliá (2010), who has reclaimed the autonomy of the historian in the investigation, documentation and interpretation of the past. The author has further argued that the treatment of evidence by a historian is different to that of a judge, a legislator or the police, who seek to impose a sentence, address a denunciation or prosecute the culprits of a crime. In Santos Juliá's view, the historian ought to make sense of the past outside of frameworks that might constraint his or her vision of the past.

Historians, though, as I realized throughout my research in Extremadura, have become the motor of broader investigations into the extrajudicial and judicial killing and disappearance of Republicans and left-wing supporters in the region. Historians' works helped many to find the name of long-gone relatives after many years of silence over their identities and fate. They have also incorporated the personal details and life story of these families and victims to particular historical studies, as mentioned before. Conversely, the testimony of those who experienced the conflict directly or indirectly and the new data emerging from mass graves have also advanced some of these studies and prompted the production of multiple regional investigations that sketch an intimate portrait of such repressive actions in local scenarios. Ignacio Fernández de Mata (2007, 202) has noted that the process that Spain has lived in the last decades has also provoked the "thematic expansion" and "democratization" of historical works, which have allowed the assimilation of other "historical subjects" that were never part of common narratives about the conflict. These works, the author further argues, have helped many families realize a long-yearned desire: to incorporate their lives in a collective history from which they had been excluded (ibid., 203). In this process of historical production, the exhumation milieu has surfaced as a space in which different forms of knowing the past coalesce, revealing the topography and idiosyncrasies of past Francoist forms of repression. In Extremadura, these actions gave place to specific political, scientific and historical realities, which gave the exhumation not only a humanitarian meaning but also turned it into a mechanism for the production of new truths about past individual and collective experiences of Francoist violence in south-western Spain.

Notes

1. See, for an example, the editorial "Spaniards at Last Confront the Ghost of Franco" in *The New York Times* (Sciolino and Daily 2002).
2. Website can be accessed at: http://www.memoriahistorica.gob.es/es-es/LaLey/Paginas/index.aspx.
3. Macé explains that the *Fundación Francisco Franco* (The Franco Foundation), an organization dedicated to preserving and promoting the legacy of the dictator, organizes still today a yearly event to commemorate the death of the dictator every 20th November. The event has a strong religious character and is attended by over 3000 people.
4. Since the beginning of the historical memory movement, the question of what to do with the monuments that celebrate the Francoist past has remained a pressing issue in political and social debates. The so-called Law of Historical Memory established in its Articles 15 the withdrawal of "coat of arms, emblems, signs and other, personal or collective, commemorative references that praise the military uprising, the Civil War or the repression carried out during the dictatorship [...], except if there are artistic, architectural or artistic-religious reasons protected by law" (Ministry of Justice 2007). Throughout the years, this has been done by some local and regional administrations but not others—as many have disagreed with the changes the legislation demands.
5. Recent institutional debates, for instance, around the fate of the Valley of the Fallen in Spain reassert this view. In 2011, an Experts Commission for the Future of the Valley of the Fallen, designated by the government of the Socialist Party (PSOE), advised the transformation of the site into a space of "shared memories" (Spanish Ministry of the Presidency 2011: 6) that transmitted the democratic values of post-dictatorship Spain.

6. This is not to say that ARMH does not have a political commitment or involvement in relation to exhumations. It is rather to point out how the main priorities of both associations have differed over the years (see Ferrándiz 2014 for an in-depth analysis).
7. Other important aims of the *Causa General* were the attribution of pensions for relatives of those who died fighting for the Francoist movement, the inscription of these victims on the Civil Registry and to obtain information about political exiles in order to repatriate them (Gil Vico 1998, 183–184).
8. Blanco Rodriguez (2007) states that depositories such as the Historical Military Service (Servicio Histórico Militar), the Civil War Section in the National History Archive in Salamanca (Sección Guerra Civil del Archivo Histórico Nacional) or the repositories of the Ministry of External Affairs and Finance (Ministerio de Asuntos Exteriores y Hacienda) were made available. Chaves Palacios (2000) also makes reference to the opening, in this period, of civil registries in local courts and town hall archives, which could not be accessed by researchers before.

References

Aguilar Fernández, Paloma. 2008a. *Políticas de la memoria y memorias de la política: el caso español en perspectiva comparada*. Madrid: Alianza Editorial.

———. 2008b. Transitional or Post-Transitional Justice? Recent Developments in the Spanish Case. *South European Society and Politics* 13 (4): 417–433.

Aguilar, Paloma. 2013. Jueces, represión y justicia transicional en España, Chile y Argentina. *Revista Internacional de Sociología* 7 (2): 281–308.

Aguilar, Paloma, and Francisco Ferrándiz. 2016. Memory, Media and Spectacle: Intervieú's Portrayal of Civil War Exhumations in the Early Years of Spanish democracy. *Journal of Spanish Cultural Studies* 17 (1): 1–25.

Aróstegui, Julio. 2009. La Ley de Memoria Histórica: Reparación de insatisfacción. *Patrimonio Cultural de España* 1: 41–60.

Bervernage, Berber, and Lore Colaert. 2014. History from the Grave? Politics of Time in Spanish Mass Graves Exhumations. *Memory Studies* 7 (4): 1–17.

Chaves Palacios, Julián. 2000. La historiografía reciente sobre la Guerra Civil 1936-1939 en los umbrales del nuevo milenio. *Anales de Historia Contemporánea* 16: 409–430.

Chaves Rodriguez, Candela. 2015. *Sentenciados. La represión franquista a través de la justicia militar y los consejos de guerra en la provincia de Badajoz, 1937-1950*. Badajoz: PREMHEX.

Chinchón, Javier. 2012. *El tratamiento judicial de la Guerra Civil y el franquismo en España. Una visión de conjunto desde el derecho internacional*. Bilbao: Deusto University.

Closa, Carlos. 2013. Spain. In *Encyclopedia of Transitional Justice, Volume 2*, ed. Nadya Nedelsky and Lavinia Stan, 459–464. Cambridge: Cambridge University Press.

Colom González, Francisco. 2010. El pasado en el presente. Qué hacer con la memoria de la Guerra Civil. *Res publica* 23: 161–174.

De Grieff, Pablo. 2014. Report of the Special Rapporteur on the Promotion of Truth, Justice, Reparation and Guarantees of Non-recurrence. In *General Assembly United Nations*, ed. Human Rights Council. Twenty-seventh session. Agenda item 3.

Druliolle, Vincent. 2015. Spain: Seeking Justice in Argentina. *Justiceinfo.net*. Available at http://www.justiceinfo.net/en/opinions/argentina-the-right-to-intervene-in-spain.html. Last Accessed: 25 Apr 2017.

Escudero Alday, Rafael. 2011. *Diccionario de memoria histórica: conceptos contra el olvido*. Madrid: Catarata.

Escudero, Rafael. 2014. Road to Impunity: The Absence of Transitional Justice Programs in Spain. *Human Rights Quarterly* 36 (1): 123–146.

Espinosa Maestre, Francisco. 2003. *La columna de la muerte: el avance del ejército franquista de Sevilla a Badajoz*. Barcelona: Crítica.

Etxeberria Gabilondo, Francisco. 2003. Panorama organizativo sobre antropología y patología forense en España. Algunas propuestas para el estudio de las fosas con restos humanos de la Guerra Civil española de 1936. *La memoria de los olvidados. Un debate sobre el silencio de la represión en España*, Universidad de Valladolid.

Etxeberría Gabilondo, Francisco. 2005. La exhumaciones de la guerra civil española desde una perspectiva antropológica y paleopatológica. Available at: http://www.uam.es/otros/sepal/actas/actas_files/trabajos/08_Caceres/50%20Com.39.pdf. Last Accessed: 25 Apr 2017.

Fernández de Mata, Ignacio. 2007. El surgimiento de la memoria histórica. Sentidos, malentendidos y disputas. In *La tradición como reclamo. Antropología en Castilla y León*, ed. Pedro Tomé Martín, 195–208. Salamanca: Consejería de Cultura y Turismo. Junta de Castilla y León.

Fernandez de Mata, Ignacio. 2011. The Rupture of the World and the Conflicts of Memory. In *Unearthing Franco's Legacy: Mass Graves and the Recovery of Historical Memory in Spain*, ed. Carlos Jeréz-Farrán and Samuel Amago, 279–304. Notre Dame, IN: University of Notre Dame Press.

Ferrándiz, Francisco. 2006. The Return of Civil War Ghosts: The Ethnography of Exhumations in Contemporary Spain. *Anthropology Today* 22 (3): 7–12.

Ferrándiz, Francisco. 2007. Exhumaciones y políticas de la memoria en la España contemporánea. *Hispania Nova. Revista de Historia Contemporánea* 7 (71).

Ferrándiz, Francisco. 2010. De las fosas comunes a los derechos humanos: El descubrimiento de las desapariciones forzadas en la España contemporánea. *Revista de Antropología Social* 19: 161–189.

Ferrándiz, Francisco. 2011. Autopsia social de un subtierro. *Isegoría. Revista de Filosofía Moral y Política* 45: 525–544.
Ferrándiz, Francisco. 2013. Exhuming the Defeated: Civil War Mass Graves in 21st Century Spain. *American Ethnologist* 40 (1): 38–54.
Ferrándiz, Francisco. 2014. *El pasado bajo tierra: exhumaciones contemporáneas de la Guerra Civil.* Barcelona: Anthropos.
Ferrándiz, Francisco, and Alejandro Baer. 2008. Digital Memory: The Visual Recording of Mass Exhumations in Contemporary Spain. *Forum Qualitative Social Research* 9 (3 Art 35): 1–23.
Gálvez Biesca, Sergio. 2006. El proceso de la recuperación de la 'memoria histórica' en España: Una aproximación a los movimientos sociales por la memoria. *International Journal of Iberian Studies* 19 (1): 25–51.
Garzón, Baltasar. 2008. Diligencias Previas Proc. Abreviado 399/2006 V. Audiencia Nacional Juzgado Central de Instrucción No. 005.
Gatti, Gabriel. 2016. Lo nuestro como en *Argentina*: Humanitarian Reason and the Latin Americanization of Victimhood in Spain. *Journal of Latin American Cultural Studies* 25 (1): 147–165.
Gil Vico, Pablo. 1998. Ideología y represión: La Causa General. *Revista de Estados Políticos (Nueva Época)* 101: 159–189.
Golob, Stephanie R. 2008. Volver: The Return of/to Transitional Justice Politics in Spain. *Journal of Spanish Cultural Studies* 9 (2): 127–141.
González-Ruibal, Alfredo. 2007. Making Things Public: Archaeologies of the Spanish Civil War. *Public Archaeology* 6: 203–226.
González-Ruibal, Alfredo. 2009. Arqueología y Memoria Histórica. Available at: http://digital.csic.es/handle/10261/31203. Last Accessed 25 Apr 2017.
Gónzalez-Ruibal, Alfredo, Xurxo Ayán Vila, and Rachel Ceasar. 2015. Ethics, Archaeology and Civil Conflict: The Case of Spain. In *Ethics and the Archaeology of Violence*, ed. Alfredo Gónzalez-Ruibal and Gabriel Moshenska. New York: Springer.
Humlebaek, Carsten. 2004. Usos políticos del pasado reciente durante los años de gobierno del PP. *Historia del Presente* 3: 157–167.
Juliá Díaz, Santos. 1979. *Orígenes del Frente Popular en España, 1934-1936.* Madrid: Siglo Veintiuno.
Juliá Díaz, Santos (ed.). 1999. *Víctimas de la Guerra Civil.* Madrid: Temas de Hoy.
Juliá Díaz, Santos. 2006. Bajo el imperio de la memoria. *Revista de Occidente* 302, 303: 7–20.
Juliá Díaz, Santos. 2010. Por la autonomía de la historia. *Claves de razón práctica* 207: 8–19.
Junquera, Natalia. 2013. La promesa que Rajoy si cumplió. *El País*, Oct 5.
Kwon, Heonik. 2008. *Ghosts of war in Vietnam.* Cambridge: Cambridge University Press.

Labanyi, Jo. 2008. Entrevista con Emilio Silva. *Journal of Spanish Cultural Studies* 9 (2): 143–155.

Labanyi, Jo. 2009. The Languages of Silence: Historical Memory, Generational Transmission and Witnessing in Contemporary Spain. *Journal of Romance Studies* 9 (3): 23–35.

Lázaro, Julio M. 2012. Garzón vuelve al banquillo por haber investigado los crímenes franquistas. *El País*, Jan 24.

Leizaola, Aitzpea. 2006. La antropología a pie de fosa. Diálogo con Francisco Etxeberría y Francisco Ferrándiz sobre la memoria de la Guerra Civil. *Ankulegi* 10: 33–46.

Macé, Jean-François. 2012. Los conflictos de la memoria en la España post-franquista (1976–2010). Entre políticas de la memoria y memorias de la política. *Bulletin Hispanique* 114 (2): 749–774.

Ministry of Justice. 2007. *Ley 52/2007, de 26 de diciembre, por la que se reconocen y amplían derechos y se establecen medidas en favor de quienes padecieron persecución o violencia durante la guerra civil y la dictadura.* http://leymemoria.mjusticia.gob.es/cs/Satellite/LeyMemoria/es/memoria-historica-522007. Last Accessed 16 Aug 2017.

Ministry of the Presidency. 2011. *Informe: Comisión de expertos para el futuro del Valle de los Caídos.*

Nora, Pierre. 1989. Between History and Memory: Les Lieux de Memoire. Special Issue: Memory and Counter-Memory, *Representations* 26: 7–24.

País, El. 2012. La ONU arremete contra el juicio a Garzón por investigar el franquismo. *El País*, Feb 10.

Preston, Paul. 1994. *The Coming of the Spanish Civil War: Reform, Reaction and Revolution in the Second Republic.* London: Routledge.

Preston, Paul. 1999. La historiografía de la guerra civil española: de Franco a la democracia. In *Tuñón de Lara y la historiografía española*, ed. José Luis de la Granja Sainz, Alberto Reig Tapia, and Ricardo Miralles, Madrid: Siglo XXI.

Preston, Paul. 2011. The Theorists of Extermination: The Origins of Violence in the Spanish Civil War. In *Unearthing Franco's Legacy: Mass Graves and the Recovery of Historical Memory in Spain*, ed. Carlos Farrán-Jerez and Samuel Amago, 42–68. Notre Dame, IN: University of Notre Dame Press.

Reig Tapia, Alberto. 1984. *Ideología e historia: sobre la represión franquista y la guerra civil.* Madrid: Akal.

Richards, Michael. 2011. Grand Narratives, Collective Memory and Social History: Public Uses of the Past in Postwar Spain. In *Unearthing Franco's Legacy: Mass Graves and the Recovery of Historical Memory in Spain*, ed. Carlos Farrán-Jerez and Samuel Amago, 121–148. Notre Dame, IN: University of Notre Dame Press.

Rodriguez, Blanco, and Juan Andrés. 2007. La historiografía de la guerra civil española. Hispania Nova. *Revista de Historia Contemporánea* 7 (741).

Rosenblatt, Adam. 2015. *Digging for the Disappeared: Forensic Science After Atrocity, Stanford Studies in Human Rights*. California: Standford University Press.

Rubin, Jonah S. 2014. Transitional Justice Against the State: Lessons from Spanish Civil Society-Led Forensic Exhumations. *The International Journal of Transitional Justice* 8 (1): 99–120.

Rubin, Jonah S. 2015. Aproximación al concepto de *desaparecido*: reflexiones sobre El Salvador y España. *Alteridades*, Memoria social. Estudios y contribuciones antropológicas 25 (49): 9–24.

Ryan, Lorraine. 2016. Memory, Transitional Justice, and Recession in Spain. *European Review* 25 (5): 1–12.

Salas Larrazábal, Ramón. 1977. *Pérdidas de la guerra*. Barcelona: Planeta.

Sciolino, Elaine and Emma, Daly. 2002. Spaniards at Last Confront the Ghost of Franco. *The New York Times*, Nov 11.

Silva Barrera, Emilio. 2003. *Las fosas de Franco: los republicanos que el dictador dejó en las cunetas*. Madrid: Temas de Hoy.

Todorov, Tzvetan. 2000. *Los abusos de la memoria*. Madrid: Taurus.

Torrús, Alejandro. 2016. Los jueces pueden tomar declaración a los 19 altos cargos franquistas a pesar de la negativa de la Fiscalía. *Público,* Oct 6.

Viejo-Rose, Dacia. 2011. *Reconstructing Spain: Cultural Heritage and Memory After Civil War*. Brighton: Sussex Academic.

CHAPTER 3

Visions of War and Postwar History in Extremadura

Recent works of Spanish historiography have spoken at length about the urgent need to engage with an alternative history of the Spanish Civil War and the Franco regime. Authors such as Alberto Reig Tapia (2006) have argued that historians today play a crucial role in dismantling what he has called the political and historical "myths" of Francoism. According to Reig Tapia "the propaganda of the Civil War has been so intense that the historiographical effort to overcome so many ideological justifications has to be, necessarily, equally intense and constant" (ibid., 21). Other historians, who also support this view, have identified further problems with historical writings about the conflict (see Preston 1999; Chaves Palacios 2000; Blanco Rodriguez 2007) and the revisionist revival some of these theses have enjoyed in the last years (see Espinosa 2005; Rodrigo 2004). Underlying the work and intentions of these scholars is a wish for a change of paradigm, which reconsiders past studies in the light of new analyses and in relation to data and sources that have emerged from the depth of official archives and other repositories.

Michel Foucault (1972) observes in his *Archaeology of Knowledge* that the formation of new discourses within a particular field, in this case that of history, has to be comprehended in relation to the conditions of their existence. Such a discursive field, he claims, needs to be understood within its limits, and in terms of the correlations it bears with other statements and the statements that it excludes (ibid., 28). Indeed, contemporary historians have linked the development of a Spanish historiographical

Z. Aragüete-Toribio, *Producing History in Spanish Civil War Exhumations*, World Histories of Crime, Culture and Violence,
DOI 10.1007/978-3-319-61270-6_3

tradition about the war to the effects of different political periods on the discipline. Since the exposure of the corpses in mass graves in the year 2000, the conditions of historiography have transformed, as the authoring of works about the recent violent past has become something sought after by many in Spain. The last two decades, as some explained to me during fieldwork, have witnessed some of the most intense production of history books about the Civil War the country has experienced. Other historians also joined associations or created special programs such as the so-called *Cátedra de Memoria Histórica del Siglo XX* (Chair of Historical Memory of the twentieth Century) in the Complutense University in Madrid (UCM), which was launched out of an agreement between two other foundations (the 1st May Foundation and the Largo Caballero Foundation). Historians have indeed acquired, whether inside of projects or as independent researchers, a concern for the social reality in which their work is embedded and this, one could say, has expanded their "system of discursivity" and filled it with new "enunciative possibilities" (Foucault 1972, 129).

This chapter examines the impact of exhumation work in the transformation of historical epistemologies around war and postwar Francoist violence, paying special attention to the case of Extremadura. In so doing, it considers how the surfacing of traces in archives and at mass graves has turned the discontinuities registered in these sources into an object of analysis for historians, archaeologists, physical anthropologists and archaeologists. Such discontinuities have become important not in order to suppress them in the elaboration of a total history of the conflict, but to discern the web of relations and events that precipitated these rearguard killings and other forms of repression (ibid.; Stoler 2010). New historical projects have developed in connection to a social demand to know what happened in the past, turning historians and scientists into active campaigners for the declassification of official files[1]—as has happened in other settings (see Da Silva Catela and Jelin 2002; Verdery 2014; Douglas 2013)—and facilitators of information in familial searches of the past, as well as activist lobbying for the recognition of victims.[2] During my fieldwork in Extremadura, I followed the work of historians and archaeologists and saw firsthand their entanglements with family groups and associations in the region. I wanted to understand how information about the war and Franco's repression was construed and constructed through their engagement with different technologies and proceedings. I examined how this practice was influenced by political and social motivations, and how these, in turn, shaped the treatment of a materiality that contains, as Derrida (1996) observes in a number of documents in Freud's archive, the sedimented violence and wounds of a censored, silenced, and beaten Republican body.

The Production of Historical Knowledge in twenty first Century Extremadura

When I asked professor Julián Chaves Palacios, historian and director of the Project for the Recovery of Historical Memory in Extremadura (PREMHEx), to describe his understanding of the widely-used term *historical memory*, he spoke of a transformation in the historiographical tendencies of the past decade and of the novel qualities that history writing had acquired in the social terrain. According to Julián, the number of works written about the violence of the war and postwar has boomed, and has dominated the market of history publications in the region in the last ten to twelve years. This extraordinary hyper-production is bound up, he explained, with the social appeal and action of civil society groups "in need of more information" (Julián Chaves Palacios, Cáceres, 2013). *Historical memory*, however, does not only refer to a form of history exegesis, but also encompasses other definitions. Julián went on to explain:

> From the historian's perspective, we have always worked with the term *memory*, always. People have added the '*historical*' adjective as a complement. I have not much to say about it but let's not get one thing wrong. When we talk about historical memory we are not only speaking about history, we are also talking about other issues. An exhumation process for instance, transcends mere research – though it is, and brings us information. It has also an important *human component*, ethical: to provide an answer to a social demand. Historical research is important but there are other matters. [Historical memory] is an important phenomenon that has taken place in the last years, but it is not only subscribed to history. History is the past but this history is providing an answer and is *demanded* by families that want dignity for their disappeared relatives. (Julián Chaves Palacios, Cáceres, 2013; emphasis added)

De Certeau (1988, 11) observed that history is as much a thing of the past as of the present, arguing that public interests and current events provide the historian with the means and context for the labour of writing. Though Julián asserts at one point, "history is the past," the connection between the production of historical texts and research and the wider social search for information about the war in recent years, as the historian implies, make the history of the conflict very much a thing of the present in Extremadura. This idea is strengthened by the fact that, in the last decade, the project has had the economic support of regional institutions. This, according to Julián, is a necessary condition that makes the historical and exhumation research programme possible today—though it is not exempt from manifold criticisms on the part of civil society groups engaged in the historical study of the past, as will be seen in later chapters. Moreover, that certain collectives in fact *demand* history—or demand to know—has fostered proximity between historians and civil society members and given place to other forms of evidence-gathering in the study of the repressive past. Hence, Palacios identifies in the fragment above how exhumation practice has also become a site of historical investigation, through the petitions of families and associations looking for the bodies of the missing.

The reading of the absent body in archives and files is complemented by anthropological and archaeological readings of the body in the mass grave, as well as the understanding of relatives, activists, and historians alike. Outside of the project, this interest in the historical investigation of war and postwar phenomena has also led to the emergence of new historical interpretations, propelled by families' own research, enthusiasts of the subject in and outside of associations, and members of small communities that emerge as local experts and amateur historians of the war in their specific geographical areas. The convergence of these groups opens up a line of inquiry into how indeed exploration into the origin, or the genesis of violence and bad death is performed and produced by each group, and also how this exploration is determined by past remains as well as present realities. Not only the work of PREMHEx, but also of other associations and individuals that engage with historical research activities, reconfigure the archaeologies of history (ibid.) already in place, its discourses and practices and the research technologies employed in the study of the repression in the region.

PREMHEx is the result of a collaborative agreement between the Regional Ministry of Culture, Badajoz Council, and Cáceres Council and the University of Extremadura (UEX), initiated in 2003. It was one of the first memory projects to be supported by a regional government (led at the time by the regional branch of the Socialist Party) in the country.

Hence—according to some of its members—it was a pioneer in creating an institutional infrastructure for the work on exhumations and historical investigation. The project is hosted by the Department of History of the regional University of Extremadura (UEX), in the city of Cáceres. From the start and until 2012, it also had a Historical Memory office in the town of Mérida, where petitions for exhumations were dealt with. These petitions normally relate to the search for those who disappeared and were violently killed, especially in the Francoist rearguard—though exhumations of Francoist supporters killed by Republicans have also been carried out. Historians and archaeologists work together with Julián Chaves Palacios on the research into archives and other depositaries, the exhumation of mass graves, and the collection of oral testimonies from survivors, direct and indirect witnesses, and family members. Throughout my time in Extremadura, I could also appreciate the special emphasis placed by members of the project on the dissemination of information through conferences, seminars, books, and articles that aimed, as I was told on many occasions, to "*revert* this historical information back into society," as archaeologist Laura Muñoz Encinar stated in an interview in 2012.

In addition to this, there is also a clear preoccupation with the quality of the data collected and its interpretation. As Julián observed in our interview, the project aims to document those unknown aspects concerning, in particular but not solely, Francoist forms of violence, and to convey this information from—in his words—a "scientific perspective." As such, there is a stress on the way information is obtained and treated, analysed and written, obeying the precept of "scientific rigour and accuracy" (Julián Chaves Palacios, Cáceres, 2013). Methodology and, in particular, researchers' discursive outputs are guided by an idea of *truth* and facticity, influenced by the deceitful and concealed nature of some evidentiary sources and their analysis in official dictatorial attempts to write the history of the contest. Additionally, their work is clearly influenced by a long tradition of scientific objectivity, which has influenced history, as well other disciplines (see Daston and Galison 2007).

This attention to the "faithful" retelling of the past is partly related to the type of data encountered in incomplete state files, where much information recorded about political sentences and executions has been skewed by state agents that contributed to the institutionalization of violence in the new Francoist State of 1939. "Rigour" and "accuracy", on the other hand, imply a wish for objectified knowledge, for a reconstruction of the past driven by the dictums of evidence and distanced from the type of ideological rhetoric that many historians identify in earlier and present works (i.e., texts of a strong left-wing ideological slant or a revisionist character). Such an objective vision ultimately "aspires to knowledge that bears no trace of the knower—knowledge unmarked by prejudice or skill, fantasy or judgment, wishing or striving" (ibid., 17). In the research into such a thorny history, the arena of knowledge production becomes a disputed and murky terrain since, for many—as Lorrain Daston (1991, 93) has remarked—facts "are robust in their existence but opaque in their meaning." Nevertheless, as seen in later chapters, such discourse and practice for "objectivity" are complex endeavours in constant negotiation with the everyday emotional and political demands of the exhumation.

Over the years, the project's thematic focus has been on the "events related to the death, disappearance, prison or exile of people from Extremadura [...] as well as concentration Camps, disciplinary battalions or penitentiary colonies (in the region during the war and after, in the postwar years of *franquismo*)" (GEHCEx report, II Encuentro Historiográfico 2007, 4). State and family archives of papers and photographs drive the process of inquiry, offering official and personal details about the person killed. These archival traces are simultaneously—where possible—scrutinised in the light of firsthand testimonies of those who experienced the violence of the conflict, those related to the missing, and other indirect accounts. Mass graves contain the ultimate material substantiation of the violence captured in the archive and the oral record, through the concreteness of the corpse and the marks inscribed on the bones. Camps, prisons, and work battalions are rich vestiges of knowledge for researchers as their formation elucidates the post-conflict detention system and handling of political detainees.

These are all sources of scrutiny that serve the historian in inferring the events, which took place in the past (Collingwood 1946, 251). They form part of the discipline's evidentiary protocols (ibid.), but are also determined by what Engelke (2008, 5), in his critique of Collingwood, has termed as "the competing pressures and regimes" within the profession and—in this case, I will add—the socio-political and legal milieus that encompass it. The information produced by the project coexists at all times with associations' rights and recognition campaigns for the status of those who lost the war. Within the context of the regional memory associations, historical data and material remains become identifiers and proof that can support claims for the legal acknowledgement of the victims of Francoist crimes during and after the conflict. In such a way, these concrete artefacts of historical meaning-making enter a different evidentiary regime (Crossland 2013), defined by the modes and protocols of the judicial and legal fields. The use of these human and material remains expands from the realm of the academic into other areas of social action, revealing different historical epistemologies under construction. The making of history in Extremadura is hence determined by the interplay between these evidentiary artefacts and regimes and their understanding and use by civil and state actors.

Activists' associations with which I met and collaborated, such as the Regional Association for the Recovery of Historical Memory in Extremadura (ARMHEx) in Badajoz, the Association for the Memory of Castuera Concentration Camp (AMECADEC) in the district of La Serena, and the Association for a Memorial in Cáceres Cemetery (AMECECA, previously PROMECECA) work closely with information from the archive and oral testimonies in order to document their rights and memorialisation campaigns. These associations often count local historians and law experts among their members and promote investigations into to the politics of memory surrounding archives, the official recognition of war and repression sites in the region, and the moral reparation of families that endured forms of political subjugation during the war and dictatorial period. The emergence of these organized groups has created an intense social network of actors that compiles, exchanges, and channels the historical information on the conflict. Within these associations, the collection of historical data is intended to address the systemic neglect and forgetting of these issues in the country. The way in which civil registries and historical and military archives are found has activated many of these claims.

For instance, in connection with the deficiencies of civil registries, it is widely stated by some of these groups and their representatives that many of the people killed without a trial or sentence died not only physically but also legally, as the causes and dates of these deaths were never fully recorded after the war or during the transition. According to some sources (Espinosa 2009), even though the decree 67 of the 10th November, 1936, allowed families to inscribe these casualties and disappearances already during the war, individuals were generally coerced into disguising the causes of death of the victims in order to secure forms of economic support later on, such as widow's pensions, or to ensure future opportunities for their offspring in public programmes such as the military service (ibid.). Many of the descendants I interviewed during fieldwork, however, often assured me that their predecessors, normally mothers, never attempted to obtain their spouse's death certificate due to the state of fear and distress in which they lived. Others refused to complete death certificates attributing a false cause to the death of their relatives. In the case of official governmental national and municipal archives and military sources, one of the main issues with which associations contend, in the present, is the persistent problem of access and declassification of administrative and judicial files, and of historical documents held in private collections of organizations such as the Francisco Franco Foundation or the Falange's archive,[3] to name just two examples. In these campaigns, which closely relate the figure of the missing with their identities in paper files of public and institutional avenues, the archive presents itself as a device of evidence accretion, in which information is read against the archival grain in disparate truth-seeking efforts.

Placing the Archive(s)

In 2006, Amnesty International Spain denounced, in their report *Victims of the Civil War and Franquismo: The Disaster in the Archives, the Privatization of Truth*,[4] the poor condition of military and municipal depositories, demanding the assessment, cataloguing, and reordering of the repression files by the Spanish state. The document was produced in the light of the Interministerial Commission for the study of the situation of the victims of the Civil War and Franquismo, undertaken in 2004. It called for the modification of the Regulations of State Archives, dated 1901,[5] and the elaboration of a Law of Archives (*Ley de Archivos*) that would enforce the management and preservation of many files that had been damaged, that had disappeared, or been classified, and which contained information about war trials, executions, and imprisonments during and after the conflict.

According to the report, produced whilst the restorative Law of Historical Memory of 2007 was being drafted, until that date, access to these records was reduced and often complicated by the confusing archival organization and arrangement of files, and the "arbitrary access criteria" (Amnesty International Report 2006, 8) used by personnel in charge of their supervision. This, on many occasions, required long waiting periods, sometimes months and years, on the part of any person seeking to obtain documentation (ibid.). Through their appeal, the organization advocated for the public and immediate availability of these documents to researchers and especially to families and survivors, who, unable to understand the peculiarities of the archival system, often had to enlist the assistance of third parties like historians or specific associations. According to Amnesty, having these papers ready for use allowed collectives affected by the violence of the war and the Franco regime to retrieve information, which "[could] prove the severe violations and abuses of human rights committed [in the past]" (Amnesty International Report 2006, 7). In the line of Amnesty's paper, documents are thus turned into the objects of "public proof" (Latour 2005) in a legal–political rights discourse and procedure. They are so, first, due to their value as potential items for moral reparation and economic reparation claims. And second, for their capacity to pin down the efficacies of past dictatorial statecraft.

The presence or absence of files containing information about disappearances and killings and their administration in the present also needs to be understood in connection to the type of repression exerted at different moments during the conflict and post-conflict. In his report to the Central Court of Instruction no. 5 of the Spanish National Court about the state of war-related historical and judicial sources in the country (in support of families' appeals to judge Baltasar Garzón in 2009), historian Francisco Espinosa (2009) explains the relation between different repressive strategies and the traces they left in local and national annals. According to the author, in the first year of the war, Francoist executions were backed by War Proclamation Orders (*Bandos de Guerra*), which at a national level provided these extrajudicial killings with a pseudolegal character (ibid.). Little is known about how these *bandos* operated at local level, according to Espinosa (2009). *Bandos* and local extrajudicial killings left thousands of deaths unaccounted for, with no death transcript in civil registries. Numerous cases were recorded as deferred inscriptions until the 1990s, though with unclear or skewed descriptions about what led to the individuals' death. For instance, many of these deaths were described as the consequence of "a collision with the armed forces," "a result of a *bando de guerra*" or, on other occasions, "as a consequence of the Glorious National Movement" (the name given to the military uprising). Nonetheless, most of these deaths have not been yet fully quantified, as ongoing research discloses new figures progressively—for instance in recent works by doctoral students such as those working for PREMHEx. Civil registries in judicial archives and municipal repositories hold information about some extrajudicial killings, but not all. They are a source for the analysis of the unbridled violence carried out during and after the conflict for historians and, in addition, archaeologists that work in the clandestine mass graves where these bodies were often buried.

From 1937, many executions were realized through court-martial procedures (*Consejos de Guerra*) and their sentences, in an effort to legitimize and institutionalize the elimination and incarceration of political prisoners and, after the war, guerrilla militias, until 1945. In comparison with the often evasive death records in the archive, resulting from extrajudicial killings, the recorded summary trials reveal the workings of a rising military jurisdiction, in which extensive information was included about suspects. Espinosa (2009) further identifies another repressive period that lasted from 1945 well into the 1950s, when the last remains of the guerrilla resistance were severely suppressed. Some authors (Aguilar 2013, 285) have also identified 13 deaths by court-martial—four by strangulation or *garrote vil* and nine by firing squad—between 1958 and 1975. The death penalty was also part of the ordinary justice model in the same period, where 41 verdicts were issued (ibid., 290). Files produced in relation to these court-martial procedures are found in depositories under the auspices of the Ministry of Defense and the Ministry of Culture, and offer an insight into the effects of the intertwining systems of military and ordinary justice in the creation and maintenance of the Francoist state (Aguilar 2013).

The complex judicial and police apparatus at the core of the emergent regime generated an exorbitant number of documents from trials and investigations instantiating a convoluted system of archives. Court-martials and their pronouncements form part of a collection of documents produced by the so-called Territorial Military Courts (*Tribunales Militares Territoriales*) and local Military Courts. According to the 2006 Amnesty International report, these archives often enclose sentences and procedural surveys containing additional information such as books, personal letters, or retrieved records from political parties and other possessions confiscated from the detainee (Amnesty International Report 2006, 8). Different territorial dispositions and jurisdictional areas of implementation composed these Territorial Military Courts. There were five main territories of jurisdiction.[6] At the same time, each Territorial Military Court covered a number of autonomous communities or regions, relying on other Military Defense Courts at local and provincial levels to conduct their rulings (ibid.). For instance, the First Territorial Military Court, whose headquarters was located in Madrid, managed the cases and sentences from Extremadura as well as from areas such as Castilla-La Mancha, Murcia, Madrid, and Valencia. Nonetheless, some of the information about the region of Extremadura is held between the General Military Archive in Madrid and Ávila's Military Archive. In addition to these archives, Amnesty International also identifies as an important vestige the archival selection of the Court of Exchequer (*Tribunal de Cuentas*), which holds dossiers about concentration Camps and work battalions, their expenses and invoices; the ample photographic and documentary fund at the Guardia Civil Archive (*Archivo de la Guardia Civil*); and documents held at the Historical Municipal Archives (*Archivo Histórico Municipal*) of distinct provinces around the country (ibid.).

To these collections we should add documents that resulted from other legal decrees and proceedings from 1939 to 1945 and after this, records generated by institutions that monitored opposing political behaviour or dissidence. Among the measures taken to reprove political affiliation during and after the war were the Law and Court of Political Responsibilities (1939), whose retroactive sentences—until 1934—involved extreme incarceration penalties, professional disqualification, fines, expropriations, and even the exile of the detainee to other villages, towns, or regions.[7] In the same years, other laws and tribunals comprised the actions of sometimes-mixed (military and ordinary) judicial structures created in the consolidation of Franco's state. The Law for the Purging of Public Employees (1939) or the Special Court for the Repression of the Masonry and Communism (1940) are examples of this. In addition to this, also in 1940, the *Causa General* was created to investigate crimes perpetuated by Republican militias and sympathizers, generating abundant information until 1960, which was often used to start new judicial trials (Aguilar 2013). Most of these judicial causes against political suspects were supported with dozens of documents seized from regional archives, left-wing Republican parties, unions, and private citizens. These have been held at the General Archive of the Civil War in Salamanca[8] since 1996.

At a later stage during the dictatorship, other institutions were created to secure control and enforce ideological and political repression during the regime's modernizing stage. The Public Order Court (*TOP*), created in 1963, is a representative paradigm, administered in the beginning mainly by civil judges (Aguilar 2013, 289). Much of the information produced by these institutions is today distributed throughout different official archives, such as the General Administration Archive, the General Military Archive in Madrid, or the General Archive of the Civil War in Salamanca, to cite a few. The ensuing report published by the governmental Interministerial Commission in the summer 2006 on the state of archives,[9] which partly answered Amnesty's demands, made apparent, through the numerous archival sources it cited, the dispersion of some collections, hinting at the taxing experience of researching the footprints of these repressive institutions.

With the enforcement of the restorative Law 52/2007 or the Law of Historical Memory, files from the National Historical Archive (where the papers of the *Causa General* are held), the General Administration Archive, the Historical Memory Documentary Centre (home to the General Archive of the Civil War) and others were digitized, and thus much data was made public online. Although some say the conditions of these repositories around the country gradually improved, especially after the passing of the aforementioned law, they did not improve radically. According to Espinosa's 2009 report, military sources, for instance, were then still chaotic. This issue also applies to the civil registries and local court records in which incomplete and inaccurate death certificates elicit the open-ended absences triggered by extrajudicial executions. As a bureaucratic tool for the public classification of citizens, the registry awards official existence to individuals in the ledgers of the nation-state. For many, especially families, the absences found in these ledgers connect these sources with past histories of loss and uncertainty, of revoked legitimacies and social anxiety. The inconsistent and tenuous files symbolize the negative representation and floundered individuation of the defeated, which was perpetuated gradually after 1939.

These gaps and silences in the registry have been the subject of much social and academic interest in the last decade. On the one hand, in recent years, historians have engaged in producing lists of names and figures that give clarity on the issue of such covert deaths, aiming to recompose an intelligible narrative of the confounding historical evidence. On the other hand, the predicaments presented by inscriptions of those killed during the war and the postwar in civil registers became the leitmotiv of protests on the part of associations demanding the completion of these repositories with the names of those never listed. This required a change in the legislation—a reform of the Civil Registry Law of 1957—that permitted other ways of attesting the causes of these individuals' deaths.

Before the present Civil Registry Law was approved in 2011, these inscriptions were limited to family members and were time-consuming and costly, requiring the testimony of two witnesses that could confirm when and how the person died. For many relatives wanting to register people who had perished in the context of the conflict, this was an arduous task. The long temporal distance between the events and the time of registration meant some relatives could not see the process through or locate witnesses, who, if still alive, might be willing to testify about the killings. After a persuasive campaign led by Andalusia-based associations (e.g., CGT [General Confederation of Labour] or *Todos los Nombres*) and other national collectives (e.g., ARMH)—with the slogan: "All victims of franquismo in thecivil registries!"—the law enforced in 2011 made inscription protocols more flexible. Now, town halls (as well as relatives) can register these deaths and witnesses are no longer needed. As the regional association ARMHEx in Extremadura explains on their blog, proof of killings has been *softened*, as registries now accept any type of evidence through which "death can be rationally inferred" (Law 20/2011 of Civil Registry, Head of State, *Boletín Oficial del Estado*, 2011, 81498). Here *soft* evidence refers to those marks, accounts, or remains from the past that no longer offer a direct experience of the conflict and require, just as the papers, files, and photographs of archives, inferential interpretation. The indexical character of the evidence, which mediates the past and "establishes a fact in a situation of uncertainty" (Csordas cited by Crossland 2013, 125) gains prevalence in the process of registering these violent deaths.

Similarly, the files from summary proceedings in court-martials have also been subject of intense controversies. Legal experts and different associations today demand the dissolution of sentences pronounced by Franco's military jurisdiction, due to the disingenuous nature of the accusations and trials performed. For many civil collectives, much of the information generated by the proceedings should be recognized as illegal, contesting its evidentiary character and reaffirming the invalidity of these sentences. These groups argue that this ought to be contemplated in the text of the Law of Historical Memory of 2007—which considers the trials and sentences illegitimate but not unlawful (Ferrándiz 2011). Such archival materials gain significance when they come into contact with these different motivations and with the making of history itself. Through them history thus acquires, as Steedman (1998, 66)—recalling Le Goff—argues, an active role as a device, a "technology of remembrance" in the construction of a social memory and in the subjective imagination and experience of the past in the present.

Excavating the Repression Files

Researchers from PREMHEx and independent historians work closely with the documents of the above-mentioned civil registries, municipal, state, and military court archives, as well as other documentary sources of relevant analysis (e.g., biographies, letters and personal scripts). Among these different files, death certificates and trial sentences bear an intimate connection to the space of the mass grave. The non-existent or incomplete documentation in civil registers and the remaining execution edicts in other state judicial repositories often trigger an image of the displaced body of the missing in furtive burial grounds, both for the researcher and for relatives and activists that engage with these records. The archive, as Carolyn Steedman (1998, 75) observes evoking Bachelard, is a space that allows for dreams and daydreams, in this context, of the violence that transpired in the local and familial scenarios of the conflict. For the third and fourth generations of historians that work in the study of archival texts in PREMHEx, the relation between these objects and the dead is metonymic: it speaks about the repressive project as a whole from the moment of the military occupation in 1936 until the postwar years in the two provinces. For other emerging local and provincial researchers, they also constitute a reminder of the episodes that took place in particular villages and towns.

In mapping these events, the historian becomes an archaeologist of books and drawers, folders and charts, imagining events and tracing sequences in order to interpret the paradigms of civil and military confrontations. In so doing, the historian's work unpacks these files and also places them in the hands of those who actively search for information in official repositories about the missing—whether relatives, activists or fellow researchers—driving these files into novel contexts of reception. The circulation of archival papers carries with it imprints and the signs of past violence. As a space that mobilizes the mind and the body through the imagination, the archive and the documents that move in and out of it stir recondite inner feelings and fears in those who come in touch with them. Visions of the past are inextricably linked to the emotions that the content of their pages provoke and provide. One can trace the dislocated effects of the politics of the repressive order in the relationship that different people establish with documents and the motivations verbalized in their descriptions and pronouncements.

In an interview with young doctoral researcher Javier Martin Bastos, who worked at PREMHEx between 2005 and 2014, the historian explained how documents had played a crucial role in the formation of a regional database of individuals who died as a result of Francoist and Republican repression as well as in prisons during and after the war. The purpose was to create a digital search engine in which the profiles of these individuals (with names, places of death, and trials) could be located through a web device and online. In the first years of Javier's participation in the project, he engaged in the retrieval of information from all local civil registries in the province of Badajoz and the north of Cáceres. This was a lengthy job that he complemented with an additional search in military and prison archives whilst he assisted colleagues with their collection of death and prison sentences elsewhere. After a few years, Javier was given the task of compiling a "white book of the Francoist repression" (Javier Martin Bastos, Cáceres, 2013) in the province of Badajoz. This would also eventually become the theme of his PhD thesis, where all the data would be analysed and published.

Observing Javier's work, one can construe that there is a strong interest in producing the figures of the violence perpetrated by both sides of the conflict. Figures, as we will see in later chapters, are too a point of contention between the historians that research Francoist forms of violence and those that have led the more revisionist currents in the country over the past decades. As quantifiable evidence, numbers acquire particular relevance in different academic and non-academic contexts, as they become raw data for accountability allegations and in public debates about the identity of victims and perpetrators. Their value and attraction resides in their capacity to strengthen both distinct historical arguments and the status of the historical knowledge being produced (Jordanova 2000, 95). For Javier, accounting for these deaths is also a way of addressing the information contained in the *Causa General*, which documented the number of deaths generated by Republican forms of repression. Javier situates this number between 1800 and 1900 individuals and estimates the number of dead as a result of Francoist violence to be around 11,500–12,000 in Extremadura alone, from 1936 to 1945. Remembering these numbers with some hesitation, due to the volume of cases recorded and in the absence of his notes, Javier's words bring out the incertitude caused by the immensity of the job and the conditions of the archive:

> I remember separate figures right now. The number of deaths by irregular execution, which is nearly a final figure, is around 9,500. People who died as a result of capital punishments were around 1,700. 800 people died in prison and 200 to 300 died for other various causes: poisoning, beatings and ill treatment and deaths after prison. And finally we have around 200 disappeared. People we don't know what happened to them. We have, for instance, documents that show the transfer of a prisoner to another prison and after that, there is no more information anywhere about him or other prisoners whose file says 'released under the custody of the Civil Guard' and there are no more records about what happened to them. Some researchers have previously interpreted these as executions—however we don't have enough data to confirm this. In other occasions, we have evidence through the testimony of families that some of these individuals were in fact executed, as we compare the details we have from the provincial prison, what is in other history books and the testimony of the prisoner's family. (Javier Martin Bastos, Cáceres, 2013)

For the historian, civil registers cannot be viewed in isolation and ought to be considered in conjunction with oral testimonies and past historical works by local historians, amateur writers, or people that have inventoried these cases locally in the past. Bearing in mind that around 50% of these executions were never registered and there are few records related to the killings, these sources provide important avenues of investigation that recount subaltern realities. In addition, the very real entanglements between these documents and the living disclose other cultural intimacies related to this kind of historical investigation. For instance, for Javier, the contact with witnesses and the account of relatives enabled him to "rethink the nature of his research" (ibid.). Personal memories from people interviewed, often accompanied by images of the missing obtained from personal collections, reminded him that the individuals on the documents were "not just names on a paper but real people" with vivid histories still attached to them (ibid.). Testimonies offered proximity to the past, according to the researcher, especially in the most advanced stages of his investigation, when the repetitive counting of thousands of cases had distanced him from the severity of the deaths recorded. This was not the case, however, at the beginning of his research, when the information contained in the archives disturbed and outraged him. The writing on these papers *shocked* him—as Stoler (2010, 181) has noted, recalling Roland Barthes in her reading of Dutch colonial files—because the files not only spoke of historical events but also about the harrowing "dramas" of some people's lives (ibid.). The feelings of distress were also incremented, according to Javier, by the physical experience of the civil registry itself, which, unlike other archives, was desolate and dusty, making working routines intense and engulfing. Death certificates and other files are embroiled with the sentiments and actions of past authoritarian pursuits, shaping the sensuous and personal encounter of the historian in the present. When these files travel from the archive and registry into the house, they enable private forms of familial reminiscence and perception.

The death certificate in Fig. 3.1 shows the way in which these documents were completed. Through a close reading of its rubric and looking to the story behind it, one can observe inconsistencies in the registration process and the frustrations these procedures sometimes cause for families. This particular record certifies the death of Libertad Gonzalez's father. Libertad is the daughter of José Gonzalez Barrero, a well-known figure in the historiography of the province, for his role as the socialist town mayor of the village of Zafra, in Badajoz, at the time of the Second Republic. Her father, Libertad remembers, was arrested in the village of Castuera on his way back from Madrid when the war had ended. After being imprisoned in a concentration Camp built in the outskirts of Castuera, he was taken out by a group of neighbours from Zafra and later executed on the way to his home village (see map of Extremadura for locations). José Gonzalez's body was never found. In a conversation with Libertad, she explained how for some years her family did not know whether he was dead or alive.

Her mother would learn that José had been killed back in 1939 through hearsay, after talking to different people in Zafra and Castuera. Years went by without news about his whereabouts. In the silence and austerity of the postwar years—Libertad recalls that her mother talked about the past to her from an early age—she "knew something bad had happened to the family" (Libertad Gonzalez, Zafra, 2011). Knowing that he had been killed in the vicinity of the village, the family inscribed José's death in the Civil Registry of Castuera in 1980, during the transitional years and after Franco's death. As shown in Fig. 3.1, this record contains details about José's birth date and place but scarce information about when and where he died. There is no a concrete date, month of death, or burial location indicating where his body was inhumed. In addition, the section dedicated to the cause of death states: "violent death due to man's direct action as a consequence of the Civil War." Even though his death was inscribed already during the democratic

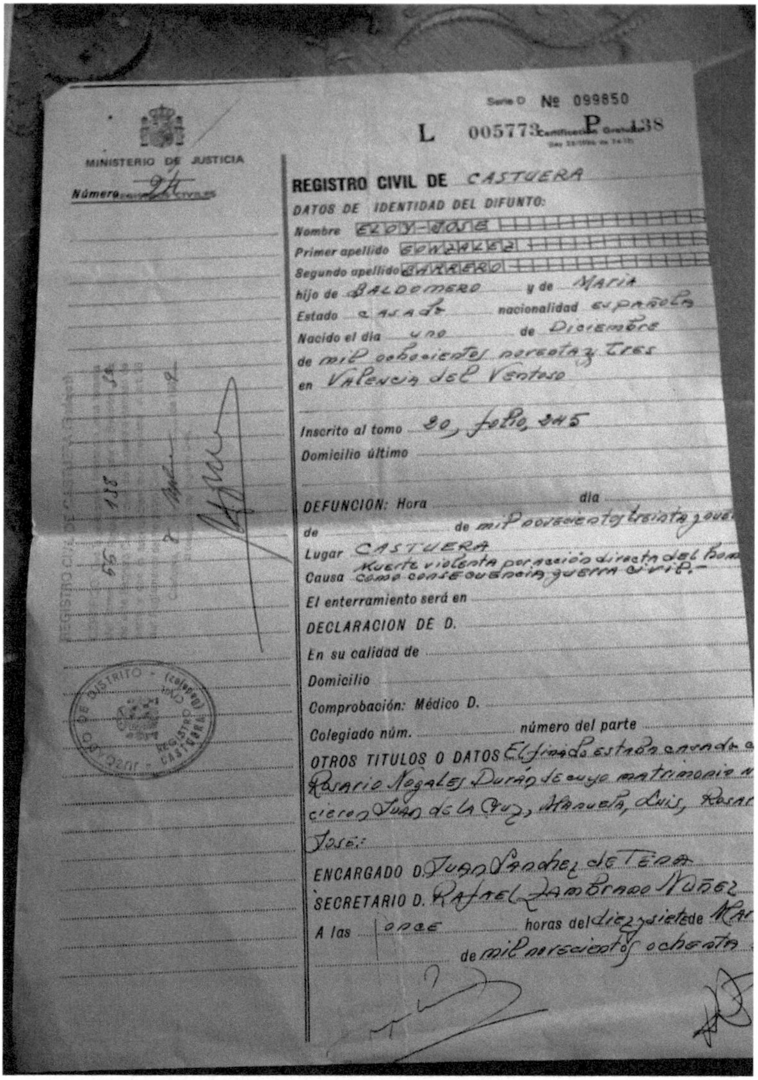
MINISTERIO DE JUSTICIA

Número

Nº 099850

L 005773

REGISTRO CIVIL DE CASTUERA

DATOS DE IDENTIDAD DEL DIFUNTO:

Nombre ELOY-JOSE

Primer apellido GONZALEZ

Segundo apellido BARRERO

hijo de BALDOMERO y de MARIA

Estado casado nacionalidad española

Nacido el día uno de Diciembre

de mil ochocientos noventa y tres

en Valencia del Ventoso

Inscrito al tomo 20, folio 245

Domicilio último

DEFUNCION: Hora día

de de mil novecientos treinta y nueve

Lugar CASTUERA

Causa Muerte violenta por acción directa del hom... como consecuencia guerra civil.-

El enterramiento será en

DECLARACION DE D.

En su calidad de

Domicilio

Comprobación: Médico D.

Colegiado núm. número del parte

OTROS TITULOS O DATOS El finado estaba casado c... Rosario Nogales Durán de cuyo matrimonio n... cieron Juan de la Cruz, Manuela, Luis, Rosar... José.

ENCARGADO D. Juan Sánchez de Tena

SECRETARIO D. Rafael Zambrano Núñez

A las once horas del diecisiete de Mar... de mil novecientos ochenta

Fig. 3.1 Death certificate of Eloy José Gonzalez Barrero, killed in 1939 and inscribed by his family in March 1980, civil registry of Castuera, Badajoz. Courtesy of Libertad González Barrero

years, it was still then attributed to the civil confrontation and no mention was made of the illicit character of the execution as an act of political repression. This deferred inscription did count, since it had the presence of two witnesses, in this case, "two right-wing neighbours," Libertad recalled, who confirmed that José Gonzalez had, in fact, been murdered.

A decade ago, Libertad met local historian José Maria Lama, who was writing a book about the war in Zafra and had great interest in José Gonzalez and his socialist mandate before and during the contest. With his research, Lama had been able to locate many files related to the life of the town mayor but also to his death. He had found, among other important records, a different certificate for the death of Libertad's father in Zafra's Civil Registry. The historian passed the file on to Libertad, thus untangling parts of the family's history that had never been known before. The certificate stated that her father had died in 1947 and not 1939. It also showed that José was a labourer and not the town mayor of the locality. The inscription, possibly completed by the local judge or a public notary during the postwar years and filled in with false details about the identity and death of the political leader, made Libertad distraught. For decades, her family, and especially her mother, had been oblivious to the existence of these records and the image they portrayed about their relative. Describing the deceiving depiction of her father in the transcript, Libertad protested: "He was already dead, they had already killed him and they still wanted to humiliate him even more?" (Libertad Gonzalez, Zafra, 2011).

Libertad sees in these distorted details about her father's death a way of dishonouring his persona and the memory of her kin. It makes her immediately recall a childhood and adolescence of public discrimination in the postwar village community. This she associated with the problems she faced in gaining access to her local school or the fact that her name was changed as an infant to Rosario by civil registry officials during the dictatorship—for Libertad, meaning "freedom", epitomized Republican ideals for Francoist authorities. The certificate, as a bureaucratic product of the dictatorial order, embodies the power of the sovereign over the life and death of José, over his body and the trails of his political persona. Notably, however, it also signals an ongoing command over or haunting (Gordon 1997) of his surviving family. The contact with such forms of familial consciousness in the present revives the file's repressive efficacy and capacity to encumber individual trauma. These sentiments are part of reciprocal exchanges between relatives and historians—as Javier implied—where memories are constructed by relying on data found by the expert and transmitted knowledge and private files of the witness and survivor.

The ramifications of Francoist sovereignty are especially visible in the files of summary trials and other judicial sentences performed by court-martial and special tribunals, where the individual is depicted through the accusations of state prosecutors, the words of the defender, and the statements of witnesses gathered in the form of public complaints, behaviour reports from local authorities (the town mayor, Civil Guard, and priest), or individual declarations. In Extremadura, two historians from PREMHEx concentrated on the study of judicial sentences that punished political affiliation to left-wing parties and unions in the years of the war and the postwar period. These two doctoral researchers are Candela Chaves and Inés Belén Fernandez, who worked closely with archival information in state military and administrative archives. Candela examined court-martials and summary trials of Republican detainees, whilst Inés studied the files of those affected by the Law of Political Responsibilities (1939)—enforced after the war to prosecute those under suspicion of having cooperated with the Republican regime.

The documents in court-martial trials for instance, as Candela explained to me, elucidate a form of repression until then undocumented in relation to Franco's military justice. These files not only included the final sentence (with resolutions like prison penalties or execution by firing squad) but also provided access to an extensive array of files that revealed why different people were condemned, how the process was initiated, what the steps were, the impressions of the prosecutor and defender, and other intrinsic details about the judicial protocol. According to the researcher, the 8000 cases identified—although not a final number—have allowed the project to "expound the Francoist cleansing process" and its meticulous reach in every village, town, and city of the province of Badajoz. Candela observes that the information in these files has to be carefully read and interpreted, as it is often "biased and inquisitorial, where accusation witnesses, pleas and declarations are given priority over those of the defence" (Candela Chaves, Cáceres 2013). Although Candela explained that she had not been able to work with very many oral testimonies from families or prisoners, she recognizes that those she managed to compile were "illuminating" when deciphering "the darkness of Francoist military justice" (ibid.). Working with these "cold files" (as she termed them) requires, in her view, the voice of those who experienced these processes to contrast the conniving character of the trials and award a "real" dimension to the proceedings (ibid.). These files are thus seen as artefacts in need of association with the subjective experience of those who lived the events recorded, to alleviate the bitterness of their existence.

Documents such as José Gonzalez Barroso's death certificate or the files of these trials and sentences also enter other spheres of social, political, and legalistic action that provide them with additional meanings in the present. For instance, the death certificate, and summary trial dictums are concomitantly an important part of the group of papers that families and survivors can collect in order to obtain a certificate of moral recognition from the Ministry of Justice. These certificates, according to the Ministry, are a form of acknowledgement, through which "Spanish Democracy honours those who were unfairly subject to persecution or violence during the Civil War and the Dictatorship" (quoted from José Gonzalez Barroso's certificate in Fig. 3.2). These documents began to be issued as a result of the Law of Historical Memory (or Law 52/2007), in an effort, on the part of the government, to acknowledge, in a legal but nevertheless subtle way, the status of these individuals as victims of the repressive Francoist system. Since then, associations such as ARMHEx in Extremadura have helped descendants like Libertad to acquire a declaration from the government (see Fig. 3.2).

These lengthy and convoluted procedures, however, require the knowledge of those used to dealing with the bureaucratic proceedings of the Spanish legal system. For many associations like ARMHEx, it is somehow paradoxical that the state does not provide easily accessible juridical help to facilitate the proceedings. To this, one has to add that searching through these documents and creating a personal history of violence can become, on occasions, emotionally onerous. Collecting these files for new purposes often means that families have to face the *fever* or *mal d'archive* in the documents—to recall Derrida's words—impregnated with the perverse reasoning of repressive orders. Nonetheless, for Libertad Gonzalez, receiving the recognition of the state was gratifying, even though one of the things she lamented was the fact that her mother was not alive to see it. She wished all of this had happened earlier, as she believed that "all homage and recognition should have been enjoyed by [her] mother", who, she recalls, never stopped thinking about her husband's fate.

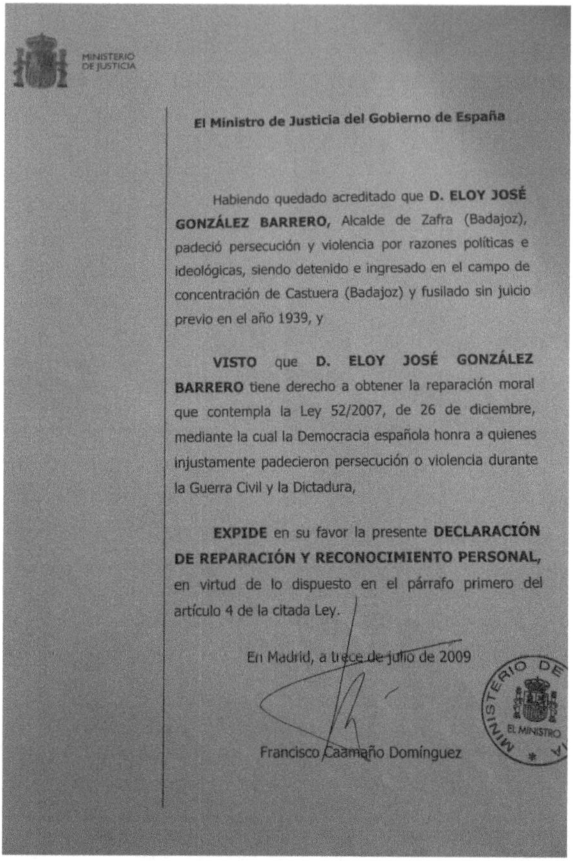

MINISTERIO DE JUSTICIA

El Ministro de Justicia del Gobierno de España

Habiendo quedado acreditado que **D. ELOY JOSÉ GONZÁLEZ BARRERO**, Alcalde de Zafra (Badajoz), padeció persecución y violencia por razones políticas e ideológicas, siendo detenido e ingresado en el campo de concentración de Castuera (Badajoz) y fusilado sin juicio previo en el año 1939, y

VISTO que **D. ELOY JOSÉ GONZÁLEZ BARRERO** tiene derecho a obtener la reparación moral que contempla la Ley 52/2007, de 26 de diciembre, mediante la cual la Democracia española honra a quienes injustamente padecieron persecución o violencia durante la Guerra Civil y la Dictadura,

EXPIDE en su favor la presente **DECLARACIÓN DE REPARACIÓN Y RECONOCIMIENTO PERSONAL**, en virtud de lo dispuesto en el párrafo primero del artículo 4 de la citada Ley.

En Madrid, a trece de julio de 2009

Francisco Caamaño Domínguez

MINISTERIO DE JUSTICIA EL MINISTRO

Fig. 3.2 Moral recognition and reparation declaration. Courtesy of Libertad González Barrero

Figure 3.2. Translation:

The Ministry of Justice of the Spanish Government

It has been accredited that ***MR ELOY JOSÉ GONZÁLEZ BARRERO****, mayor of Zafra (Badajoz), was subject to persecution and violence for political and ideological reasons, having been detained and jailed*

in the Castuera concentration camp (Badajoz) and executed without prior trial in 1939 and

***ACKNOWLEDGED** that **MR ELOY JOSÉ GONZÁLEZ BARRERO** has the right to obtain the moral reparation contemplated under the Law 52/2007, passed in 26 December, through which the Spanish Democracy honours those who were unfairly subject to persecution or violence during the Civil War and the Dictatorship,*

*[This Ministry] **ISSUES** on his behalf this **REPARATION AND PERSONAL RECOGNITION DECLARATION** by virtue of that stated in the first paragraph of article 4 of the law in question.*

In Madrid, thirteen of July 2009,

Signature

History-production endeavours have provided the documents encountered in official and personal archives with many social lives. They have become part of individuals' personal collections, where they become props for memory recall (Hirsch 2012; Murphy 2011; Trundle 2011). Through other acts of compilation, they have entered present institutional regimes where they evidence the persecution and killing of the defeated. In their use, the event of the killing is interpreted time and time again, as an object of historical exegetical writing, a token in the intimate retelling of personal histories, or evidence of a family's tragedy in the eyes of the democratic state. The information contained in their pages represents the marks of the necropolitical order (Mbembe 2003) deployed by the dictatorial enterprise, which superintended the deaths of the defeated and fostered continuing forms of oppression through their exclusion or condemnation in the archive. Upon the encounter with the relative, activist, or historian, the criminal vision of the subject promoted by these death certificates and military sentences acquires other shades and undertones. Searching in the archive becomes, as Steedman (1998, 73) has highlighted, a "process of identification" and "individuation" that aims to devise the historical identity of the dead through the familial, political, or scientific deciphering of its papers. The space of these archives is inseparably woven with other processes of identification performed by the archaeologist in the physical space of the mass grave. Here the lists of missing individuals compiled by the historian, the military trials, and oral testimonies are contrasted with the information inscribed on bones and objects and their archaeological interpretation. In the construction of historical knowledge about the conflict, the site of the mass grave emerges as a different place of collection and recollection. To understand the flows of information production about the past in the region, one has to engage with a multi-sited vision of the archive that also considers the materiality and relational properties of the exhumation site as an integral part of the process of historical inquiry.

Exhumations as Historical Research

In Extremadura, the first exhumation of the twenty first century took place in the Mina de Valdihuelo between the villages of Alburquerque, San Vicente de Alcántara, and Villar del Rey in the province of Badajoz in 2003. In the exhumation of the mine, 16 bodies were recovered—70 years after their deaths—by a team of archaeologists and volunteers and also with the help of historians. This exhumation marked the beginning of more than a decade of archaeological excavations for the regional PREMHEx. The exhumation in the Mina de Valdihuelo took place before the project had officially been created and stands as an example of an early endeavour influenced by the rise of the exhumation movement nationwide. Relatives of the missing, as elsewhere, have demanded these exhumations ever since in Extremadura. To accomplish them, they have relied on both the project and its archaeological experts, but also on the work of other independent teams hired on an ad hoc basis by historical memory associations.

In this section, I will concentrate mainly on the exhumation work undertaken by PREMHEx and their understanding and performance of mass grave excavations. During 2011 and 2012, I collaborated closely with their team, attending different prospections[10] and the localization and exhumation of human remains. As well as being framed by the goals of the research project, these processes are also bound by the idiosyncrasies of regional and state laws and the political interest they incite. Exhumation processes have undergone different stages in the last decades, marked especially by fluctuating governmental support. As already mentioned, the uncovering of bodies of the defeated is not free of controversy or adverse reactions at local, regional, and national levels.

For PREMHEx, while exhumations have been driven by families' appeals to recover the human remains of their relatives, excavations also provide them with materials, which allow for a different interpretation of the past. As archives illustrate the Francoist imaginary through textual manifestations of violence in documents, the discovery of the body in the mass grave offers a raw image of alternative stories of death and disappearance. Cayetano Ibarra, the exhumations coordinator at PREMHEx at the time, whose work consisted in compiling families' demands and initiating the investigation and location of the mass graves, explained to me that exhumations are crucial in order to document unrecorded episodes of repression in the archive. Cayetano's collaboration with the project stemmed from his previous involvement with the *Junta de Extremadura* (*Government of Extremadura*), where he held other positions as part of the administration. He was also the socialist (PSOE) town mayor of his home village, Fuente de Cantos (Badajoz) in the '90s, and the author of a detailed book about the history of the conflict in his locality. His implication in the project relates to both his personal interest in writing the history of the war and his family's experience of Francoist repression marked by his grandfather's killing. For the coordinator of exhumations, mass graves are inevitably enmeshed in a project of historical investigation because they contribute to "elucidating other versions of the history that the dictatorship never told" (Cayetano Ibarra, Badajoz, 2013). Mass graves then become revealing, and as such, become the object of historical and archaeological methodologies in the research undertaking. From the project, they are carefully examined in connection to an established. Far from being a unified set of recommended guidelines prescribed by a national official entity, the protocol followed by PREMHEx was designed by the regional project, drawing on their knowledge and training and on their own work on mass graves over the years.

Some have considered the absence of a centralised protocol—that is, until 2011, when the state finally approved one—a reflection of the lack of commitment to exhumation ventures on the part of the government. For years, teams have mostly worked according to their own investigative modus operandi, informed by the goals of the actors (whether associations or projects) leading the mass-grave search. Protocols like the one employed in Extremadura—similar to those used by other teams nationally and internationally—involve previous historical research in archives for information about the detentions and executions; the gathering of oral testimonies about the killings; the search and location of the mass grave area; securing exhumation permits from local authorities or private land owners; the exhumation and identification of the human remains and objects in the grave; the elaboration of reports about the findings that could eventually be read by families and other audiences; and, finally, the reburial of the corpses.

For some archaeologists and expert practitioners (see Gassiot and Steadman 2008), the disengaged position of governmental actors in the regulation of scientific work around mass graves and thus, in the creation of a suitable and cohesive protocol, means that exhumation processes can often be hindered by the antagonistic positions of local official bodies towards the investigation of these war and postwar sites (ibid.). According to Gassiot and Steadman (2008, 434), this is what their team experienced in Catalonia, where political opposition subtly hampered the development of their work on various occasions. Moreover, Francisco Ferrándiz (2011, 538) has remarked that the protocols established in different autonomous communities, often heterogeneous and uneven, have "ordered excavations" without clarifying crucial aspects of the work, such as their "juridical regime" (ibid.; Montero 2010).

In 2011, the socialist government that enforced the Law of Historical Memory in 2007 approved a national exhumations protocol, a few months before the end of their mandate. Based on the international 1991 UN exhumation guidelines (*El País* 2011), this measure nevertheless arrived eleven years after the first exhumation had taken place, with the purpose of providing an accredited protocol for those regions still without one. Indeed, the problem that some of those involved in the exhumation of mass graves have with governmental dispositions is not solely a concern with the creation of a state-crafted set of standards. Instead, it has more to do with the general unwillingness of state elites to fully endorse the unearthing and study of these past crimes judicially and as a historical project. Archaeologists such as Alfredo González Ruibal (2009, 110) have commented critically that by eluding the responsibility of implementing, overseeing, and administering exhumations nationwide—and instead leaving these procedures to families—the state has failed to contemplate exhumation work as a "truly investigative labour", which is part of a long term effort to create a lasting collective memory of the conflict (ibid.). It seems that the state's hesitation and vacillation towards the recovery of these bodies are founded on the unease evoked by their prominent bio-presence and by what these corpses represent in political and social terms.

Governmental rulings have had a decisive impact on the way these scientific projects have been accomplished in recent years. For instance, in Extremadura, Cayetano Ibarra described how exhumations have undergone different periods linked to the support and funding received from local and national administrations. During the first period, dating from the beginning of the project until 2007, he explained that it was the regional Ministry of Culture who mainly backed exhumations. Although it did not have a specific budget for "historical memory activities," it contributed to specific excavations because there was a "vocation to help" (Cayetano Ibarra, Badajoz, 2013). Agreements were also signed with local town halls, so that financial aid could reach them for the coordination of infrastructure related to the exhumation project. The second period, which ran from 2007 to 2011, was marked by subsidies provided by the national Ministry of the Presidency, as a result of the Law of Historical Memory of 2007. These subsidies were available to family groups and associations in order to promote and facilitate exhumations, rendering them accountable for the application process and the administration of the grant and project—including the search for the archaeological team.

In Extremadura, families and associations often rely on PREMHEx—as well as other associations like ARMHEx—to help with these bureaucratic and financial procedures, as well as to solve other practical issues such as the attainment of permits from the regional Heritage Office or the hiring of an archaeological team. In Extremadura, exhumations are subject to heritage laws. This adds another layer of complexity to the planning of the excavation, as the law understands these sites in the same way as pre-historic sites and does not regard them as a matter of urgency. Often, the delay experienced due to such bureaucratic processes would cause much exasperation in families and associations (see Chaps. 4 and 5). As with the previously noted certificates of moral recognition, the funding projects from the Ministry of the Presidency were hard-won operations that needed the guidance of those versed in the language and praxis of state forms. According to Cayetano, many of the applications filled in without advice often failed to obtain funding. The abstruse and slow nature and tempo of some of these bureaucratic procedures can have, on occasions, a direct impact on the way people live the process—as shown in later examples—on their hopes and expectations, negatively marking the experience of searching for such long-absent corpses.

The latest period, which runs from 2011 until today, is associated with the dismantling of funds from the Ministry of the Presidency effected gradually by the right-wing government of the Popular Party (PP) since the general election of November 2011. Regional and local elections held in May that same year also gave the victory to PP in many local constituencies around the country. For groups involved in the excavation of mass graves, this meant a return to the beginnings of the exhumation venture. Extremadura was governed between 2011 and 2015 by the conservative PP, and Cáceres Provincial Council did not support the agreement that made PREMHEx possible at the start. This, Cayetano assured me, made things more complicated, as there was not the same will to exhume in regional governmental frontbenches. Exhumations carried out in that period, according to the PREMHEx coordinator, have been accomplished thanks to the team of volunteers that collaborated with the project under the supervision of the project's archaeologist and physical anthropologist, Laura Muñoz Encinar. These recourses in fact saved money in the process, as then but also today families no longer receive financial aid from the Spanish state.

During fieldwork, I collaborated on exhumations that in all cases had secured funds from the Ministry of the Presidency. In two of these exhumations located in the villages of Castuera and Puebla de Alcocer, in the province of Badajoz (discussed in Chaps. 4 and 5), the grant allowed for the search for and identification of human remains and their return to the families, but also for an exhaustive analysis of these sites as spaces of acute historical value—especially for the project and its team members. This was also the case in the example of the mass grave in the village of Zorita, in the province of Cáceres, analysed in Chap. 7. Nonetheless, here the remains were never found, inspiring other actions of historical enunciation. Certainly, these political, economic, familial, and academic relations with the past shape exhumations in Extremadura. As Paola Filippucci (2010, 78) has observed in the case of Great War remembrance in France, "a keen consciousness of temporality and keen sense of historicity" determines the way in which some groups remember the past and project it onto both the present and future.

In contrast to the hesitant attitude of different governments towards the investigation and commemoration of Civil War and postwar deaths caused by Francoist repression, the historical work carried out in Extremadura is fuelled by a wish to make the past public, by a kind of "*historia magistra vitae*" (Koselleck 2004, 26), which aims to exemplify the experience of past generations for those who did not live the conflict, and which is fuelled in turn by a filial desire to restitute the identity—whether political or not—of the missing in public and official discourses. Decentralized efforts to remember and study the past emanate from an aspiration to contest an abounding instrumental silence and forgetting. The exhumations led by PREMHEx in Extremadura are at once a locus where political intricacies at different levels are played out and a place for the construction of new historical imaginaries. Just like the archive, the exhumation site enlivens the dreams and daydreams of its participants, who weave a profuse vision of the conflict through empirical and emotional understandings of its materiality and technological treatment.

Exhumation work follows the scientific drive of the institutional project and is deeply entangled with the work of the historian. Archaeologist and physical anthropologist Laura Muñoz Encinar, director of exhumation activities between 2005 and 2014, trained as a historian and sees the exhumation as the last step in the process of documentation—from the archive to the grave—in the study of war and postwar forms of repression in the region. Her work is intimately connected to the research of other project members like Javier or Candela, and also to the studies of local historians in the places where mass graves are found. Working on the exhumation of these mass graves involves contrasting different sets of data provided by the files obtained in repositories, the accounts of witnesses, and the content of the unmarked grave. As Laura observes, the scientific handling of these mass burial sites aids the interpretation of those repressive files such as death certificates, incomplete lists, prison registers, and the like, which on many occasions "do not illustrate the reality" of the executions and extrajudicial acts of violence (Laura Muñoz Encinar, Fregenal de la Sierra, 2011). The materials found in the clandestine burials created during the war and after are constantly cross-referenced (Latour 1999) in a dialectic exercise between the archaeological object and the archive, to shed light on the death mechanisms and repression tactics used by the perpetrators.

As Laura explained to a group of families and neighbours in a commemorative act in October 2011:

> To commence the research activity [of the mass grave] we need to produce those lists in which we try to find out the birth date of these people and their death date—which on many occasions does not correspond with the real execution date. [We try to discover] the conditions and the causes of death, since we see how those conditions registered in the archives […] do not correspond at all with the facts that the scientific analysis of the remains provide us with. For instance, sometimes we find in the archive deaths due to '*clash with the public force*'. [But through the corpse] we can see that this is not real. (Laura Muñoz Encinar, Fregenal de la Sierra, 2011)

Deriving from this view is the idea of the exhumation space as a site of information production. For Muñoz Encinar, archaeological praxis and physical anthropological analysis can bring important knowledge "about the identity of repressed victims and also [help] to discover facts about the repression carried out in the area of study" (ibid.). The aim of the identification and individuation of the bodies is hence twofold. It consists not only in learning the names of those in the grave but also in situating them in a historical context, "to find out how they were murdered, in which moment, and to know what happened around the time of their deaths and in the course of the repressive process" (ibid.). Exhumation research thus entails a detailed methodological approach in which the excavation and documentation of these remains is meticulously conducted. Trained in the past as a member of high-profile research teams dedicated to the excavation of pre-historic sites such as the famous *Atapuerca* settlements in northern Spain, Laura's management of these sites is exhaustive and influenced by the her previous professional experience. A careful probing of the terrain and thorough recording are used during each excavation phase to extract substantial information from the burial site. Her methodology was also connected to her work as a PhD researcher studying Francoist sites and modes of repression in Extremadura through mass grave exhumations.

As Daston and Galison (1992) have observed, the painstaking technical procedures used in the gathering and interpretation of bountiful information are part of a scientific effort to elaborate a form of knowledge that is objective and impartial—part of the research goals of the project. In this context, the scientific method is employed to serve the analysis of these materials, which could be used as judicial *hard* evidence, in future truth-seeking structures of national or international reach—as the archaeologist pointed out on several occasions. In this juncture, the way in which evidence is made visible acquires a significant interest, as the excavation process unveils the idiosyncrasies of another system of information collection—composed by the archaeological handling, classification, and taxonomy of human remains and their objects. From the in-depth analysis of materials in the field, and later in the laboratory, where bones and objects are classified and inventoried, the materiality of the exhumation site speaks through means of scientific lexicons and hypotheses that animate the interpretation of the past. As Laura explained about her own archaeological practice:

> When we find the mass grave, we are going to investigate it in reverse order. We are going to remove the soil and document every event that took place in that deposit from the moment we find the grave backwards. We do this through a vertical reading, a stratigraphic reading of the soil and through a spatial reading of the mass grave. Once the mass grave has been excavated we are going to geo-reference all the objects and the bodies. We are going to see where they are, how they are positioned, the relationship each body bears with the rest and how each body and object are related. We do this in order to reconstruct tri-dimensionally the mass grave and find out how the bodies were buried, how they got there. These bodies, through their objects, provide us with information about who they are, what objects they have, and why. We have to ask why a person dressed in one way and not other, for instance, in order to find out their social status; if they have valuable objects or not, to know whether they were in prison and registered; if they have other significant objects that can point out concrete information, such as pencils—which tell us the literacy degree of that person—or lighters, objects related to the person's habits. There are certain objects that are going to give us information about the traits of the individuals. However, those objects and corpses that we have geo-referenced and analysed through archaeological methodologies from a global perspective also help us to understand the characteristics of the group and their repression *experience*, going beyond the mere identification of the bodies. (Laura Muñoz Encinar, Cáceres, 2012; emphasis added)

In Fig. 3.3, one can see this methodology and taxonomy in practice. On the sheet, part of the anthropological report elaborated by the archaeologist after an exhumation, the photograph of the corpse in the field coexists with pre-mortem information extracted from its bones and its scientific illustration. Objects are separately considered in an archaeological record of the mass burial site. As elucidated by the example and words of the researcher, once cleaned and restored, bones and objects enter into a process of interpretation in which the age, sex, and pathologies of the skeletons are observed in connection with the cultural and social attributes of the individual, provided by the artefacts they carry. The global study to which the archaeologist refers in this quote encompasses a comparative view of the exhumation space. Such a vision associates the characteristics of each single individual to the traits presented by the rest of the group and to the nature of the deposit or burial itself. These aspects are then considered in connection with the social history and the material vestiges in the repressive landscape of the region.

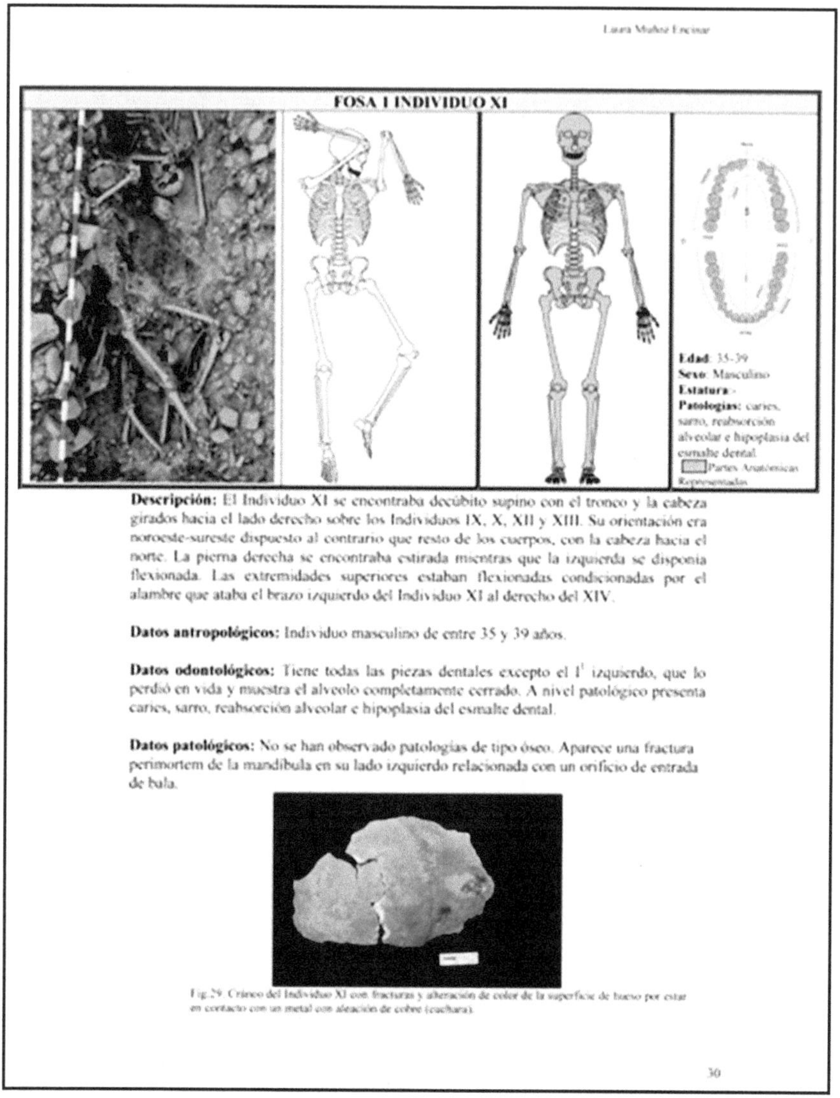

Laura Muñoz Encinar

FOSA 1 INDIVIDUO XI

Edad: 35-39
Sexo: Masculino
Estatura: -
Patologías: caries, sarro, reabsorción alveolar e hipoplasia del esmalte dental.
Partes Anatómicas Representadas

Descripción: El Individuo XI se encontraba decúbito supino con el tronco y la cabeza girados hacia el lado derecho sobre los Individuos IX, X, XII y XIII. Su orientación era noroeste-sureste dispuesto al contrario que resto de los cuerpos, con la cabeza hacia el norte. La pierna derecha se encontraba estirada mientras que la izquierda se disponía flexionada. Las extremidades superiores estaban flexionadas condicionadas por el alambre que ataba el brazo izquierdo del Individuo XI al derecho del XIV.

Datos antropológicos: Individuo masculino de entre 35 y 39 años.

Datos odontológicos: Tiene todas las piezas dentales excepto el I[1] izquierdo, que lo perdió en vida y muestra el alveolo completamente cerrado. A nivel patológico presenta caries, sarro, reabsorción alveolar e hipoplasia del esmalte dental.

Datos patológicos: No se han observado patologías de tipo óseo. Aparece una fractura perimortem de la mandíbula en su lado izquierdo relacionada con un orificio de entrada de bala.

30

Fig. 3.3 Example of the anthropological record of an individual (*Individuo IX*) found in Mass Grave 1 in the village of Castuera, Badajoz. The sheet contains a description of the position and orientation of the body in the mass grave, anthropological details (age, gender), and details about the individual's dental and pathological conditions. There is also a close up image of the individual's skull and fractures. Courtesy of Laura Muñoz Encinar

This approach is influenced by archaeological currents favouring a relational approach to the study of conflict sites. In the same way, Laura's study of the mass grave seeks to relate this prime site of repression to other spaces of violence such as the prison or the war front, in order to allow for the construction of a diachronic and integrated vision of the conflict (ibid.). This treatment of the mass grave is also determined by a growing trend in archaeological circles to consider the so-called archaeology of memory or conflict archaeology—led in Spain, among others, by archaeologist such as Alfredo González Ruibal (2012; see also Crossland 2012; Schofield 2008). The interspersed perception of the materiality of the conflict places the work of Laura at the core of a history-making exercise, but also at the core of an endeavour to recognize these sites as part of the traumatic collective heritage of the contemporary past (Buchli and Lucas 2001) in Spain. As the archaeologist asserts, through this praxis the initial premise that mass graves exist can be proven, even though many people deny their actuality still today. Exhumation research is hence envisaged as a practice with the function of "make[ing] a social identity explicit" (De Certeau 1988, 45) through knowledge generated about the violent past.

Indeed, this purpose is in line with the overall focus of the institutional project and with the goals of the social movement for the recovery of historical memory. Nonetheless, the scientific interpretation of these bodies and their objects is understood differently in the socio-political arena in which they exist. This can be appreciated throughout the exhumation process and, finally, in the reburial and memorialisation of the human remains and their belongings. In Extremadura, for instance, the reburial is often—but not solely—performed collectively, especially since DNA identification is usually complicated due to the degeneration of the bones in the acidic soil of the region. Other issues, such as the impossibility of finding relatives to obtain suitable samples for identification, make the task of individuation arduous. In most of the exhumations I followed, family and activist associations opted for a group burial and commemoration, emphasizing their significance as symbols of collective remembrance and political reclaim. Likewise, the post-exhumation treatment of the objects encountered in the mass grave evokes a similar social response. For instance, many families who find their relatives choose to donate their personal effects to the provincial museum with a desire to attain a form of public avowal, as Laura explained in an interview. In other cases, and as I discuss in Chap. 7, their storage in the museum is a contentious issue—especially for intermediary associations who promote exhumations but which might not have direct kinship links to the bodies—since the regional patrimony law requires these objects to be deposited in the provincial repository in the absence of a living relative.

Conceived of and enacted as scientific entities, and existing as part and locus of the political, legal, and familial worlds of the living, documents, bones, and objects incorporate the fragmented details about the killings in the Francoist rearguard. Their presence stimulates a history of violence, whose meanings are constantly negotiated through techo-scientific discourse and practice, political action, and social and familial remembrance. As hybrids—to use Latour's definition (1993)—which fluctuate between different epistemologies, they can often resolve or generate uncertainty, serve the purpose of political agendas, or alleviate the ongoing searches of families. In the light of the faulty knots that compose such networks of deceitful remnants and skewed politics, following different exhumation ventures can shed light on the entanglements between the official archive and the mass grave, and the effects of these objects on the individual and collective assembling of a discursive system around the history of the conflict. Similarly, as indexes of the person that once was, these human remains, documents, images and objects have a profound capacity to affect the relations and reactions that form around the event of the exhumation, as their distressed materiality meets with the traumatic experience of survivors and the personal worlds of those from different generations. The following chapters explore the intricacies of the historical project in connection to two excavations sites in different sociopolitical contexts. Throughout these chapters, the exhumation of different mass graves is treated as a central space in which the identity of the missing is co-produced through material, narrative, and affective expressions that converge during the process.

Notes

1. See the recent manifesto *El acceso a los archivos y la Memoria Histórica del siglo XX* (Access to Archives and Historical Memory in the twentieth Century), compiled by the Chair of Historical Memory of the twentieth Century in 2014, which reclaims the need and importance of opening all official repositories to the public.
2. An example of these organizations is the association in the southwest of the country *Todos los Nombres* (Sevilla, Andalusia), initiated by the Association for Memory and Justice in Andalusia (MHJ) and the General

Work Confederation in Andalusia (CGT), which works to make information in archives and elsewhere accessible to the public (see their website http://www.todoslosnombres.org).

3. This information has also been contrasted in informal conversations with practitioners in the field, historians, and archaeologists working closely with these vestiges, such as Javier Martín Bastos (researcher from PREMHEx, University of Extremadura), Antonio López Rodriguez (historian and collaborator of AMECADEC), and Jimmi Jimenez (historian and archaeologist, part of the scientific group ARANZADI in the Basque Country).
4. Original title: *Víctimas de la Guerra Civil y el franquismo: el desastre de los archivos, la privatización de la verdad* (Amnesty International 2006).
5. The report suggests the re-writing of the regulations, created over a century ago, in order to adapt its guidelines to technologies available at present. One of the main requests in recent years has been the digitalization of many of these files for public download.
6. These jurisdictional areas corresponded to five different Military Territorial Tribunals: the First Territorial Tribunal in Madrid (covering the areas of Extremadura, Castilla La Mancha, Murcia, Madrid y Valencia); the Second Territorial Tribunal in Sevilla (covering the region of Andalusia and the cities of Ceuta and Melilla); Third Territorial Tribunal in Barcelona (covering the areas of Cataluña, Aragón, Islas Baleares and Navarra); Fourth Territorial Tribunal in A Coruña (covering the areas of Galicia, Asturias, Castilla y León, Cantabria, País Vasco y La Rioja); and finally, the Fifth Territorial Tribunal in Santa Cruz de Tenerife (covering the Canary Islands) (Information extracted from Amnesty International Report 2006).
7. According to Aguilar (2013) in her reading of Lanero (1996), up to 300,000 individuals had a file in the Tribunal's archive as a result of these legal actions.
8. After the passing of the Law of Historical Memory in 2007, the archive joined the collection of the newly created Historical Memory Documentary Centre, inciting requests that demanded the return of some of these seized files to the regions and archives from which they came originally. This was the case with the documents from Cataluña, confiscated from the Generalitat (Cataluña's regional government) by Francoist troops at the end of the war. In 2006, some of these files were returned to Cataluña, though most recently the region of Castilla y León claimed the unconstitutional character of the transference of the boxes. The claim was dismissed by the Constitutional Tribunal in favour of the restoration of the files in early 2013 (Constela, *El País,* 2013).
9. *Informe sobre Archivos*, Comisión Interministerial 2006.

10. A prospection consists in the examination of the land in search of the mass grave. It is the first step in the field and in the archaeological process towards locating an unmarked burial site.

References

Aguilar, Paloma. 2013. Jueces, represión y justicia transicional en España, Chile y Argentina. *Revista Internacional de Sociología* 7 (2): 281–308.

Amnesty International. 2006. Víctimas de la Guerra Civil y el Franquismo: el desastre de los archivos, la privatización de la verdad. Available at https://doc.es.amnesty.org/cgi-bin/ai/BRSCGI/Victimas%20de%20la%20guerra%20civil%20y%20el%20régimen%20franquista?CMD=VEROBJ&MLKOB=25254750202. Last accessed 25.04.2017.

Blanco Rodriguez, Juan Andrés. 2007. La historiografía de la guerra civil española. Hispania Nova. *Revista de Historia Contemporánea*, 7.

Buchli, Victor, Gavin Lucas, and Margaret Cox. 2001. *Archaeologies of the Contemporary Past.* London: Routledge.

Catela, Ludmila da Silva, and Elizabeth Jelin. 2002. *Los archivos de la represión: documentos, memoria y verdad.* Madrid: Siglo XXI.

Chaves Palacios, Julián. 2000. La historiografía reciente sobre la Guerra Civil 1936-1939 en los umbrales del nuevo milenio. *Anales de Historia Contemporánea* 16: 409–430.

Collingwood, R.G. 1946. *The Idea of History.* Oxford: Clarendon Press.

Constenla, Tereixa. 2013. El constitucional avala el envío de los papeles de Salamanca a Cataluña. *El País*, February 1.

Crossland, Zoë. 2013. Evidential Regimes of Forensic Archaeology. *Annual Review of Anthropology* 42: 121–137.

Crossland, Zoë. 2012. The Archaeology of Contemporary Conflict. *The Oxford Handbook of the Archaeology of Ritual and Religion.* New York: Oxford University Press.

Daston, Lorraine. 1991. Marvellous Facts and Miraculous Evidence in Early Modern Europe. *Critical Inquiry* 18 (1): 93–124.

Daston, Lorraine, and Peter Galison. 2007. *Objectivity.* New York: Zone.

Daston, Lorraine, and Peter Galison. 1992. The Image of Objectivity. *Representations*, Special Issue: Seeing Science, (40): 81–128.

De Certeau, Michel. 1988. *The Writing of History.* New York: Columbia University Press.

Derrida, Jacques. 1996. *Archive Fever: A Freudian Impression Religion and Postmodernism.* Chicago: University of Chicago Press.

Douglas, Lee. 2013. Los regímenes probatorios de la ciencia y la visión: la ciencia forense y la exhumación del pasado. In *Human Rights/Copy Rights: Los archivos visuals en la época de la declasificación*, ed. Cristián Gómez-Moya. Santiago de Chile: Universidad de Chile, Museo de Arte Contemporáneo.

Engleke, Mathew. 2008. The Objects of Evidence. *Journal of the Royal Anthropological Institute* 14 (1): 1–21.

Espinosa Maestre, Francisco. 2009. Informe sobre la represión franquista. Estado de la cuestión. Available at: http://www.todoslosnombres.org/content/materiales/informe-sobre-la-represion-franquista-estado-la-cuestion. Last accessed: 25.04.2017.

Ferrándiz, Francisco. 2011. Autopsia social de un subtierro. *Isegoría Revista de Filosofía Moral y Política* 45: 525–544.

Filippucci, Paola. 2010. Archaeology and the Anthropology of Memory: Takes on the Recent Past. In *Archaeology and Anthropology: Understanding Similarities, Exploring Differences*, ed. by Duncan Garrow and Thomas Yarrow. Oxford: Oxbow Books.

Fiona Murphy. 2011. Archives of Sorrow: An Exploration of Australia's Stolen Generations and their Journey into the Past. *History and Anthropology* 22 (4): 481–495.

Francisco Espinosa Maestre. 2005. Agosto de 1936. Terror y propaganda. Los orígenes de la Causa General. *Pasado y memoria* (4): 15–25.

Foucault, Michel. 1972. *The Archaeology of Knowledge*. London: Tavistock Publications.

Gassiot Ballbé, Ermengol and Dawnie Wolfe Steadman. 2008. The Political, Social and Scientific Contexts of Archaeological Investigations of Mass Graves in Spain. *Archaeologies: Journal of the World Archaeological Congress* 4 (3): 429–444.

González-Ruibal, Alfredo. 2012. From the Battlefield to the Labour Camp: Archaeology of the Civil War and Dictatorship in Spain. *Antiquity* 86: 456–473.

González-Ruibal, Alfredo. 2009. Arqueología y Memoria Histórica. Available at: http://digital.csic.es/handle/10261/31203. Last accessed 25.04.2017.

Gordon, Avery. 1997. *Ghostly Matters: Haunting and the Sociological Imagination*. Minneapolis: University of Minnesota Press.

Hirsch, Marianne. 2012. *The Generation of Postmemory: Writing and Visual Culture After the Holocaust*. New York, NY and Chichester: Columbia University Press.

Jordanova, Ludmilla J. 2000. *History in Practice*. London: Arnold.

Koselleck, Reinhart. 2004. *Futures Past: On the Semantics of Historical Time*. New York and Chichester: Columbia University Press.

Lanero, Mónica. 1996. *Una milicia de la justicia. La política judicial del franquismo (1936-1945)*. Madrid: Centro de Estudios Constitucionales.

Latour, Bruno. 1999. *Pandora's Hope: Essays on the Reality of Science Studies*. Cambridge, MA and London: Harvard University Press.

Latour, Bruno. 2005. From Realpolitik to Dingpolitik. An Introduction to Making Things Public. In *Making Things Public: Atmospheres of Democracy*, ed. Bruno Latour and Peter Weibel. London: MIT Press.

Mbembe Achilles. 2003. Necropolitics. *Public Culture* 15 (1): 11–40.

Montero, Juan. 2010. Exhumando el legado material de la represión franquista: de la percepción social a la encrucijada jurídica y patrimonial. In *Recorriendo la memoria/Touring Memory,* ed. Jaime Almansa Sánchez. Oxford: Archaeopress.

Preston, Paul. 1999. La historiografía de la guerra civil española: de Franco a la democracia. In *Tuñón de Lara y la historiografía española,* ed. José Luis de la Granja Sainz, Alberto Reig Tapia, and Ricardo Miralles. Madrid: Siglo XXI.

Reig Tapia, Alberto. 2006. *La Cruzada de 1936: Mito y Memoria.* Madrid: Alianza Editorial.

Rodrigo, Javier. 2004. Los mitos de la derecha historiográfica. Sobre la memoria de la Guerra Civil y el revisionismo a la española. *Historia del Presente* 3: 185–195.

Schofield, John A. 2008. *Aftermath: Readings in the Archaeology of Recent Conflict.* New York: Springer.

Steedman, Carolyn. 1998. The Space of Memory: In an Archive. *History of the Human Sciences* 11 (4): 65–83.

Stoler, Ann L. 2010. *Along the Archival Grain. Epistemic Anxieties and Colonial Common Sense.* Oxford: Princeton University Press.

Trundle, Catherine. 2011. Searching for culpability in the archives: Commonwealth nuclear test veterans' claimsfor compensation History and Anthropology. History and Anthropology, 22 (4): 497–512.

Verdery, Katherine. 2014. *Secrets and Truth: Ethnography in the Archive of Romania's Secret Police.* Budapest: Central European University Press.

CHAPTER 4

Exhuming the Body of the Unknown

During 2011, between 7 and 10 archaeological interventions in mass graves from the war and the postwar period took place in the southwestern territory of Extremadura. With the exception of one site, for which the regional association ARMHEx organized the excavation with the aid of an independent archaeological group, the regional PREMHEx and its archaeological team carried out all of the exhumations and mass grave searches that took place that year. In August 2011, I joined the archaeological team led by Laura Muñoz Encinar to collaborate on the exhumation of two mass graves connected to the history of a concentration Camp in the village of Castuera, located in the northeast of the province of Badajoz. The exhumation had been promoted through the advocacy work of an activist association formed by members of different generations that aimed to recover the history of the site and of the violence in the area. The following summer, in July 2012, I collaborated on a second exhumation project, where two other mass graves were unearthed in the village of Puebla the Alcocer, a few kilometres away from the first location. The exhumation in Puebla de Alcocer was organized by a group of families, who searched for their direct and indirect relatives killed and buried in mass graves.

This chapter and Chap. 5 deal with the study of these two exhumation campaigns respectively. In the analysis of the two sites, the two chapters aim to explore how social, political, and familial regimes influence scientific work and, in turn, how scientific interpretations and methods shape the imagination of the repressive event during the unearthing

Z. Aragüete-Toribio, *Producing History in Spanish Civil War Exhumations*, World Histories of Crime, Culture and Violence,
DOI 10.1007/978-3-319-61270-6_4

of the mass graves. In both exhumations, the practices of archaeology, physical anthropology, and history displayed distinct nuances and relevance, directly linked to the intentions behind each search for human remains. In the case of Castuera, discussed in the following chapter, the scientific hypotheses around the unknown corpses in mass graves gained profound relevance in relation to the scarce information surrounding these killings. The scientific intervention at the mass grave became, as Latour (1999) has observed of other scientific projects, a way to produce certainty about the historical event and to prove the existence of mass executions connected to the Camp. Uncertainty marked the careful method deployed by the archaeologist and the constant relation of the mass grave and the archive. It also marked the ways in which these corpses went from being mere bones to social beings, through scientific scrutiny and individuation and in contact with the aspirations of activists and descendents who searched for their relatives in the area.

Producing a History of the Camp

The exhumation of the mass graves located in Castuera cemetery constituted a milestone for activists and researchers who, in recent years, had dedicated extensive efforts to investigating and commemorating the war and postwar history of defeat in the village and surrounding areas. For local and regional historians and also archaeologists from PREMHEx such as Laura Muñoz Encinar, these mass burials were key for the acquisition of new data that could shed light over and corroborate the information already gathered from oral testimonies and archives about the repression in the village. Most significantly, the exhumation sought to find additional clues about the existence of a concentration Camp located in the outskirts of the village between 1939 and February 1940. The historical significance of the graves was also salient in the work carried out by the activist association who initially promoted the excavation, namely the *Asociación Memorial Campo de Concentración de Castuera* (Association for the Memory of Castuera Concentration Camp or AMECADEC). For some time, the group had worked for the public recognition and memorialisation of war spaces—such as Castuera concentration camp and other detention and war sites—as well as the histories of loss of Republicans who had been imprisoned or killed during or as a result of the conflict. According to various oral accounts and historical information gathered by local researchers, the existence of these mass graves seemed intimately connected, from the start, to the functioning of the Camp and also embroiled with the fate of the prisoners who disappeared at the site. As Laura explained in an interview in 2012, though much was already known about the repressive apparatus in Castuera, "the greatest materialization of this repression was found in the mass grave" (Laura Muñoz Encinar, Cáceres, 2012). The location of these burials then offered new avenues for the interpretation of what happened at the Camp, the repressive mechanisms used at different moments during the war, and the broader history of irregular and institutionalize violence in the area.

Renowned otherwise for its bountiful production of the infamous Spanish Christmas sweet known as *turrón* and its wool and olive oil industry, Castuera—with over 5000 inhabitants at present—was in 1936 one of the most significant enclaves of the Republican government in the midst of the war (Vila 1999; López Rodriguez 2006). When Badajoz fell to General Franco's military occupation in mid-August, 1936, the capital of the south of the region and headquarters of the Republican administration were transferred to Castuera, still under Republican rule (Vila 1999; López Rodriguez 2006). Castuera remained a site of Republican activity until 1938, the year when some of these territories fell in the so-called battle of *La Bolsa de la Serena* (The Serene Pocket)—fought between Franco's military troops and paramilitary allies and Republican forces and militia. The town's role during the first years of the war, as a locus of the Republican governmental administration and its previous convoluted history between left- and right-wing political parties during the Second Republic, is recalled in some testimonies and historical accounts as one reason for the fierce Francoist repression experienced between 1938 and the most immediate postwar years (1939–1945) in the village.

The fall of *la Serena* has become an important temporal landmark for local and regional historians—as new data keeps emerging—for understanding the development of the warfare apparatus in both Republican and Francoist flanks in southern Extremadura. Moreover, it has also become a referent in local studies of historical penitentiary arrangements—especially concerning Franco's prisons and Camps—and the formal and informal characteristics they acquired towards the end of the conflict (see López Rodriguez 2006 and contributions in the *Revista de Estudios Extremeños* 2011). For instance, the violent struggle for dominance over *la Serena* and the ensuing loss of these Republican enclaves to Franco's military and Falange ended in the capture of numerous Republican collaborators that were soon placed in different prisons, work battalions, and detention Camps. In 1939, during the last months of the combat, the disintegration of the Extremadura war front (see Hinojosa 2009) quickly gave rise to the mass displacement of countless Republican war prisoners consecrated to improvised—sometimes newly created—prison vestiges in several areas in the north-east of the province.

In this regard, the village of Castuera became a prime location for mass detention. Built between March and April of 1939 under Francoist rule, and situated three kilometres away from the village, Castuera concentration camp aimed to house the flocks of political prisoners coming from the fragmented war front and other prisons and detention sites (León et al. 2011). The Camp, as a number of local researchers told me repeatedly, was deployed as a main instrument in the redistribution of prisoners throughout the Spanish territory. Nonetheless, not all prisoners faced the same fate. Whilst some waited to be judged or to be relocated, many others—considered "the most dangerous", for their political significance in left-wing organizations—were executed and buried in the vicinity of the detention Camp. According to certain popular versions and some survivors' accounts, some prisoners were killed and thrown into the depths of the nearby mine of *La Gamonita* (López Rodriguez 2013). Others were executed on the journey back to their hometown—this was the case for Libertad's father, discussed in Chap. 3, who never arrived in Zafra—or killed and buried in impromptu mass graves dug by the roadside leading from the Camp to the village or at the rear of the village cemetery.

The Camp, however, was not a well-known site, and has never been included in historical textbooks or the social imaginary of the region. As happened in other towns, it was the work of local historians that propelled the search for more information about the site at an early stage. In Castuera, one of the first people to research the history of the Camp was historian Antonio López Rodriguez. With links to the University of Extremadura (UEX), Antonio's investigation contributed greatly to the making of the history of Francoist repression and imprisonment in Castuera and its surrounding villages. Over the years, he has also collected the names and numbers of people that were repressed, executed, and who had disappeared in these areas. In an interview with Antonio, he gave me some clues as to why the Camp was such an unfamiliar location, not only regionally but also for villagers. He spoke to me of the strong feeling of terror the Camp and the violent repressive mechanisms used on its prisoners had provoked in the population of the nearby village. According to Antonio, neighbours feared being punished by the new authorities, for any affiliation with anti-Francoist ideas under the post-occupation regime could have resulted in one's imprisonment or death. José Ramón González (2006), another historian from *la Serena*, has observed that such a disquieted atmosphere propelled the quick adhesion of the majority of the population to the values and rituals of Franco's New State during and after the conflict in the village. In Castuera, forms of extrajudicial and judicial violence were experienced during the village occupation in 1938 and after the war ended in 1939.

Moreover, historians and local researchers also relate the lack of awareness and the denial of the existence of the Camp in historical discourses to a lack of existing information about the prison compound in some of the main official military archives. In the following interview excerpt, Antonio López refers to the case of Ávila's Military Archive,[1] opened to the public and researchers in 1995:

AL: Here [in Castuera] many people denied the existence [of the Camp].

ZA: And is there information in Ávila about the Camp of Castuera?

AL: There is, but it is very fragmented. The little information there is, it's interesting because of the absences you find within it ...[For instance] there are four inventory lists (*estadillas*) [of prisoners from the Camp] from the end of July 1939 that are *correlative* (emphasis in original). This means that these lists existed before and they continued to exist after this date. However, there are none. No one has been able to find them. They should be inside that same file and they are not. They were mandatory communications sent from here [Castuera] every day at 5 pm to the chief military staff. They had to send statutory reports with the information of new admissions and casualties or relocations... Where are they?

For the historian, the military archive becomes an incomplete resource for the formation of a historical narrative—in which the fragmented nature of its files is contested (*Where are they?*)—for he admits the "temporal sequence" (Koselleck 2004) of the events recorded has been disrupted. In the case of Castuera concentration camp, Antonio López wanted to fill in the gaps of the archive in order, in his words, to promote a dynamic discourse about the Camp "which did not exist before." His aim of resolving the suspicious fractures that burden the archival narrative about the Camp led him to other sources that contested the attentive mishandling of files and fathomed the incertitude around the destiny and identity of the Camp's prisoners. Through his research, Antonio attracted the interest of those whose lives were inextricably entangled with the violence of the war, the occupation, and the detention site. Many had lost relatives during the 1938 seizure, in the course of the military and paramilitary Francoist domination. Others, from other parts of the region and indeed the country, had relatives who disappeared after being taken to prisons in the village and to the Camp. Antonio drew from these, as well as from other stories from relatives and survivors of the Camp and prisons, work battalions, guerrilla fighters, or even once-collaborators with the Francoist regime[2] in order to understand the scope of the violence at different moments in time and the functioning of vestiges such as the prisons and Camps in the area. Through looking at these life histories, Antonio gathered information that could be contrasted with that of the inconclusive archive. Conversely, through his research he could also provide traces of past detentions, found in official documents, for those families who were still looking for information about their murdered kin and the events that preceded their detention and disappearance.

Antonio López's investigation sparked the interest of a local group of neighbours from Castuera, some of who were affiliated to political parties such as *Izquierda Unida* (United Left, henceforth IU), PSOE and other left-wing organizations. Antonio and this group of neighbours would later form the association AMECADEC, legally constituted in 2006. Throughout the years, with support from families and survivors affected by the conflict, the collective became committed to promoting the historical significance of the Camp and the reparation of relatives of the missing and survivors. In an interview carried out with its then president, Guillermo León, in 2011, he described to me how the association initially emerged as "a kind of communion between these new generations and the families of repressed people who had been searching for their kin," acting as a platform through which these families could channel their demands, especially in the absence of a state-driven mechanism that could support their needs (Guillermo León Cáceres, Badajoz, 2011). Unveiling the history of the Camp was also intrinsic to their efforts and work across generations. Throughout the years, the group engaged with different activities to memorialise the Camp and remember familial stories of violence. Activities have ranged from organizing annual commemorative events inside the Camp or coordinating campaigns to protect the site, to planning and delivering history courses, didactic units for schools, or book presentations in the region. Such endeavours, following Lambek and Antze (1996, xvii), became cultural vehicles through which the memory of the detention site was made apparent. Through these, however, history-making and remembering were turned into powerful collective and dynamic expressions aimed at reformulating social ties and commitments (Lambek 1996, 239).

For instance, in the commemorative events that the association has conducted since 2006, strong messages of personal and political denouncement often filled the eroded footprints of the Camp, of which a few traits survive today, turning the space into an arena where different claims for legitimacy were enacted. The event, which comprises a pilgrimage from the main village square to the site of confinement,[3] is celebrated inside the precinct of the overgrown and deserted plain. Such events, Guillermo León observed in our interview, advocate the "social acknowledgement in the public sphere" of those who experienced direct and indirect forms of political violence, emphasizing that the association intends to provide a space of "support" and "catharsis" for families who could not mourn or utter their unsettling sentiments during the post-war years. Upon attending these events, one can observe the decidedly familial focus that the association seeks to provide. The improvised stage near the base, where a concrete Catholic cross once stood as part of the Camp's architecture, was distinctly promoted as a place for the children and grand-children of political prisoners—who died or survived—to share their life accounts (Fig. 4.1).

Michael Lambek (1996, 245) has observed in his study on memory, history, and spirit possession in Madagascar how private experiences and their mediation through narrative, performance, or material constructions can provide idioms for uttering "collective experiences and identity." In Castuera, these voices, which spoke about direct experiences of loss, were often interlaced with symbolic representations of left-wing political groups and their claims to the past. Many at these events beseeched a much-cherished Republican past, and like others in associations like the Foro, hoped for its future revival in the country's political realm. The whole range of political references and symbols, songs, and expressions, mixed with personal expressions of suffering,

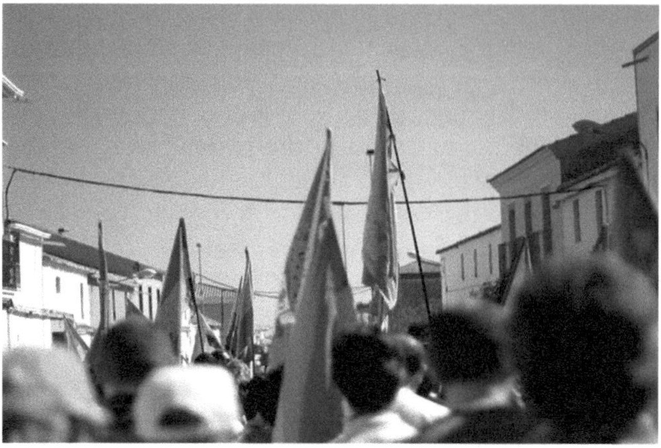

Fig. 4.1 Pilgrimage from the village to the Camp

provided the event with manifold social and historical meanings. The numerous Republican, Communist, and other flags waved, the sounds of the *Internationale* erupting from the speakers on the stage, and the use of certain Republican idioms and emblems impregnated the empty space of the Camp with the traits of past and present political identities. Together with the speeches of survivors and relatives, militants and activist voices also demanded public condemnation of these killings and disappearances and pleaded for solidarity and support on the part of present public administrations at a regional and national level. The event certainly fitted with the overall "moral" objective of the association that León had identified in our conversation. It also, however, tallied with a collective political purpose, in which past tragic stories shaped a wider appeal for historical recognition, facilitating a space in which the past could be addressed.

In 2012 the association dedicated the commemorative act in the Camp to the exhumations that took place inside the village cemetery the previous summer, in 2011. In the act, the president of the association, Guillermo León, read a manifesto in which the association openly denounced the inactive role of the state in the recovery of the human remains of the Republican missing, declaring "mass graves should have been exhumed by the Spanish State and not by AMECADEC". In León's words, as he read the manifesto, the exhumation of these corpses lays at the core of the larger struggle lived between associations, family groups, and the central government. As part of this act of public mourning, mass graves and the bodies of the war dead became symbolic of a laden "democratic integrity"—as the president remarked later in his intervention. In his words, these corpses bear the inaction of different governments in the history of the locality. The speech also addressed the resistance that some local political actors had shown towards the memorialisation of the Camp, the exhumation of the mass graves of the cemetery, and other association initiatives.

The endeavours of the association with regard to the Camp often met with antagonism from local and regional branches of different governments. During my stay in 2011, for instance, some members of the association voiced on several occasions exasperation with the scarce support received from the local governing branch of the Socialist Party over the years. Although at a regional level the socialist administration had supported and instigated the investigation and memorialisation of activities associated with the memory of the war, in Castuera, the local socio-political scenario led to a far more complex situation with the work carried out by AMECADEC. As some members and political activists angrily assured me, before the municipal and autonomic elections of 2011 that placed the right-wing *Partido Popular* (Popular Party, PP) in power—in many villages like Castuera and in the regional *Junta or Gobierno de Extremadura*—the socialist town hall had been opposed to actively backing the listing of the Camp as a Site of Cultural Interest (*Bien de Interés Cultural*) or to cultural events such as exhibitions and book publications about the Camp. In some members' views, the socialist town hall preferred Castuera to be commonly known for its *turrón* production than for the existence of a concentration Camp, hinting at the perception of the Camp as a type of "negative heritage" (Meskell 2002) in the eyes of some village neighbours and political representatives.

Similar disputes surrounded the exhumations of mass graves promoted by AMECADEC in 2010. When the association began the process of locating the mass graves with the help of the regional and institutionally coordinated PREMHEx and with a grant from the Ministry of the Presidency, the town hall requested that the association, as León explained, give their verbal commitment to *only* open the mass burials after the elections of May 2011 (Guillermo León Cáceres, Badajoz, 2011). León acknowledged that some in the ruling Socialist Party in Castuera regarded the unearthing of the corpses in the cemetery mass graves as a political risk before voting day. This, as other people agreed, was also the case in other villages in the province around the time of the regional elections. The potential presence of the bare bones awakened feelings of unease in many, as their posthumous lives were still very much entangled with the political meanings they retained from the past and which permeated the present. Corpses are, as Katherine Verdery (1999) has highlighted, "protean" and, as such, a central part of the struggle between groups aiming to offer understandings of the value of Castuera war sites. As these mass graves appeared to be the ultimate proof of a history of repression in the area, their materiality became a central point through which to articulate competing claims about the bodies' historical significance and their present place in contemporary politics.

Excavating Mass Grave 1 and Mass Grave 3

The techno-scientific search for and exhumation of the mass graves at the rear of the village cemetery, situated on the road that led from the Camp to the village, aimed to provide historical depth to the remnants of the Camp's architecture, to its fragmented memory and archival trail. In his exploration of the relation between memory and science, Ian Hacking (1996) has argued that scientific expertise can emerge as a technology for discerning the underlying truths of memory. For historians like Antonio López and researchers from PREMHEx, the scientific methodology applied to the study of mass graves opened a line of investigation through which to understand the inner workings of the Camp, but also, most importantly, the overall military strategies of the Francoist army in the area and at the nearby front. Additionally, however, these forms of "deep knowledge" (Foucault 1980; Hacking 1996) that historical, archaeological, and anthropological know-how generated, provided new concepts, classifications, and descriptions through which activist motivations and claims acquired legitimacy and through which intergenerational trauma was elucidated.

Unlike other sites that I visited later on in my research, the bodies searched for in Castuera were unknown to those who witnessed the burial, to the historian and more broadly to anyone in the village. Taking into consideration, as Antonio's historical research had revealed, that more than 12,000 prisoners passed through the Camp during the year that it was operative, and that many of these men came from other parts of the region and the country (López Rodriguez 2006, 2013), the probability of knowing to whom these remains might belong was especially narrow. When, in January 2011, location works led by Laura Muñoz Encinar brought to light the existence of nine potential mass graves scattered around the back of the precinct of the cemetery, these latent and nameless corpses became the object of scientific and activist historical scrutiny inasmuch as they triggered familial recall. Though aware of the messy reality of the repression and killings in the area, for those families in the village whose relatives' bodies remained unfound, the exhumations constituted a reason to hope for the return of the bones of their disappeared kin. The unearthing of these graves and their archaeological interpretation elicited past memories and, as Hacking (1996, 72) has observed of psychology and other memory-related sciences, served to reconstruct the inner soul of the living, who still today suffered for these war losses.

The excavation of two of the nine mass graves began in August 2011, after months of frustratingly waiting for permits from the Heritage Office—delayed due to the municipal elections of May 2011. A team formed by professional archaeologists, student volunteers from the University of Extremadura, and members of AMECADEC conducted the work under the supervision of Laura Muñoz Encinar, the leading archaeologist of exhumation projects for PREMHEx. The excavation was facilitated by the new local town hall, now led by the right-wing Popular Party (PP), with the support of United Left (IU)—to which many activists from AMECADEC were affiliated at that time. Taking into account the history of extreme friction shared by left- and right-wing parties in Spain, such a coalition could be seen as an unlikely and remote occurrence. IU's move, however, has to be understood in light of the regional politics at play during those years in Extremadura. As had happened at regional level, where IU's abstention from bestowing their votes to PSOE during the act of parliamentary investiture gave the victory to the right-wing party (Aroca Mérida for *Hoy* 2011), in Castuera, both parties governed in coalition, keeping PSOE out of the local government. The new PP town hall provided the team with storage space in the cemetery as well as some additional logistic support. This was unusual in the context of an exhumation. The PP–IU alliance had prompted a curious response from the right-wing party, which, in other places, had generally avoided and refused to support exhumation campaigns. The coalition, however, had given more headway to the association, who now benefited from some, though still very limited, support from the local government.

The two mass graves excavated, namely Mass Grave 1 and Mass Grave 3, were located near the small cemetery chapel that stood at the centre of the burial ground, which once marked the place where the old limit of the cemetery was drawn. For years, testimonies of people who visited relatives in the Camp had spoken to Antonio López about their recollection of seeing empty dug-out holes next to the cemetery wall that would be hastily covered overnight, suggesting an execution had taken place the night before. Effectively, the perpetrators of the killings deliberately placed these burials outside of the cemetery limits—as also happened in other locations around the region and the country. With the years, these dormant mass graves had been absorbed by the broadening of the cemetery boundaries in 1940 and enclosed in the community of the dead from which they had been excluded (Ferrándiz 2011).

The disposition of the mass graves contrasted with the burial of the corpses of a group of Francoist allies killed by Republican forces during the occupation in 1938, which rested in the crypt inside the same chapel. These corpses remind one of the victorious dead that revisionist rhetoric claims as the "heroes" of wartime Spain, even today, in Internet blogs and forums.[4] In the landscape of the cemetery, mass graves also contrasted with other carefully looked-after niches, adorned with flowers, candles, and individual headstones that bore the name of other village deceased. The disparity between these and the unmarked burials reminded many of the different treatment these corpses had received. In this context, scientific practice erupted in the municipal burial ground, unveiling a conflicted *deathspace* deeply embedded in distinct dead body politics (Young and Light 2012, 137). In the terrain of the cemetery, the soil was unpacked and the mass grave hollowed, in order to trace the violent event back from the moment in which the corpses were buried to the moment in which the people themselves were tortured and killed.

The internments located in Mass Graves 1 and 3 had already been connected to a repressive moment through the initial location work carried out in January 2011. As Laura Muñoz explains in the exhumation report produced for the Heritage Office after the intervention, by 2011 the different skulls and shoe soles that had been found, together with an array of objects such as "coins, fragments of fabric and a zip, a flask, a bullet and handgun bullet shells" (Muñoz Encinar 2011: 15), on the surface of Mass Grave 1 hinted at the site of an execution. Throughout the exhumation, the aim was to corroborate this initial idea through an analysis of information obtained inside the mass grave and Antonio López's data, including the testimonies he had collected over the years. When I joined the team as a member of the archaeological excavation campaign and a volunteer social anthropologist recording interviews with the families that approached the site, I quickly became versed in the meticulous methodology that aimed, as Laura explained to us and later in her report, to anticipate different variables in the mass graves, that would throw light on the identity of the skeletons and on the historical context of the killings (Muñoz Encinar 2011, 9).

The methodological approach followed was based on the principle of Harris' stratigraphic units (SU), a common method in archaeological practice, which documented the deposition of the layers inside the mass grave—since layers would provide a temporal sequence of the repressive event through their colours and textures. The stratigraphic study was combined with the recording of the spatial distribution of the cadavers and objects and their individuation (Muñoz Encinar 2011, 9). Throughout the excavation of Mass Graves 1 and 3, progressive observation of the corpses as they were uncovered was undertaken as part of a painstaking system that included the careful removal of soil, the constant photographing of the dig, layer by layer, and later, of each body and object. It also combined rigorous note-taking and drawing exercises of the space of the grave, its different stratigraphic units, and finally, of the skeletons and their positions once they had been exposed. Throughout the process volunteers were cautioned with the widely known archaeological aphorism reminding us that archaeology is a "destructive process." This became salient, especially in the absence of additional data from archives or direct relatives connected to the bodies. Moreover, in the excavation of Mass Graves 1 and 3, the bones and objects uncovered were affected by severe problems of conservation. With no other biographical information about the corpses, the act of digging, documenting, and inventorying the findings in the mass graves became decisive for obtaining information that would later condition the general interpretation of the burial sites.

The task of observation on the field became, as Lorraine Daston and Elizabeth Lunbeck (2011) have examined in the volume *Histories of Scientific Observation*, a form of scientific evidence in and of itself, determined by a method, but most importantly, by how that method was applied. Considering the precarious state of some human remains in both mass graves, the performance of daily recordings and annotations became one of the most significant tools in the study of these particular materials. As Laura told me in an informal conversation, most of her analysis in Castuera was done in situ (i.e., bone measurements or descriptions), since many body parts broke as soon as they were removed from the ground. In such a way, the mass grave became a laboratory (Latour 1999), marked by cords that carefully separated the mass grave into symmetrical squares. Each square had a letter, which helped archaeologists delineate a field of reference. Through a grid of coordinates and its classifications, archaeologists could later compress the elements of the burial site into words and diagrams in their notebooks and final reports (ibid.).

Working inside these grids was crucial, archaeologists warned us. The soil belonging to each zone had to remain isolated from the rest in order to facilitate the identification of the unknown remains. The content of each bucket was hence carefully sifted and examined separately, in case small materials had been brushed away. All bodies were to be uncovered and their contours outlined, first of all. Their exhumation would be carried out at the end. If we unearthed an object associated with a skeleton, this had to remain where it was found, as it could provide vital information about the historical context of the grave and the relation between *individuals*—as bodies were referred to in the archaeological record. Once completely disinterred, each body received a number and was given a "formalized data sheet" (Muñoz Encinar 2011, 66), in which bone measurements and descriptions were included. The mass grave and its skeletons were photographed and drawn—first on a one-dimensional gridded paper and, later, on a digital three-dimensional model, which located them in the topography of the cemetery (Fig. 4.2).

Nadia Abu El-Haj (1998) has observed in her study of Palestinian and Israeli archaeological sites how the methods and the practical logic of archaeology is often entangled with broader political and personal intentions. The care with which these mass graves were excavated, from its walls to the bones—where we were advised to use long wooden sticks to avoid causing any damage—spoke of a will to extract every possible detail that could be used as evidence of the killings. Archaeologists sought to discern the modus operandi used by the perpetrators, the chronology of the burial, and, finally, the profile of the corpses and their identities—in the event of possible DNA typing. In the final report elaborated by Laura Muñoz for the Heritage Office after the exhumation and laboratory work had been completed, the two mass graves investigated were confirmed as interments related to the Civil War (Mass Grave 1) and as

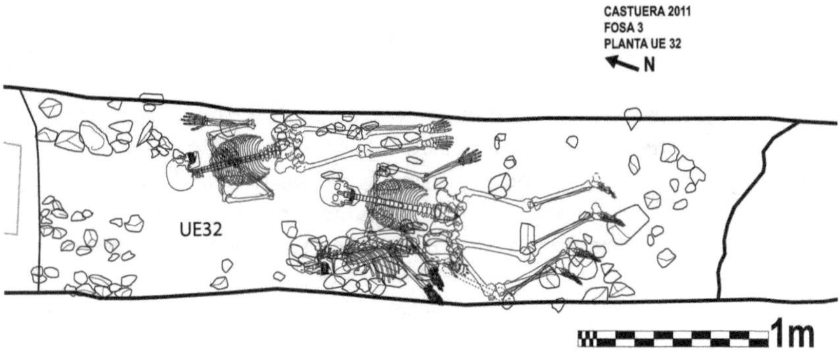

Fig. 4.2 Archaeological drawing of the human remains found in Mass Grave 3. Courtesy of Laura Muñoz Encinar

undocumented executions carried out during the first years of the dictatorial regime (Mass Grave 3). The human remains of three men were unearthed in Mass Grave 3, the first grave excavated. The corpses of another eighteen men were found in Mass Grave 1.

The group of individuals found in Mass Grave 1, as the archaeological report shows, was considered a possible "saca and execution of a group from the isolated prisoners barracks in the concentration Camp" (Muñoz Encinar 2011, 74). This coincided with similar procedures already documented in the study of the area and the detention site by Antonio López Rodriguez. Recalling the narratives given by some of his respondents, Antonio explained to me how, on many occasions, neighbours from surrounding villages came to the Camp and selected prisoners from their localities to be executed. Through testimonies, he had documented "how these repressive strategies were articulated through the making of a list by a municipal committee. Then, some came to the Camp, took prisoners, and killed them in their villages" (Antonio López Rodriguez, Castuera, 2011). Members of paramilitary groups such as *Falange* performed some of these individual and group abductions. Antonio deduced that executions would have also been ordered by a judge within the Camp's system—as occurred in other concentration Camps elsewhere. These death sentences might have been dictated as a result of a War Proclamation Order (*Bando de Guerra*), through which groups of 18–20 prisoners were killed every three days. Antonio found some files containing these sentences; nonetheless, according to the historian, there are still scarce records of the proceedings (Antonio López Rodriguez, Castuera, 2011).

As the extension of the burials was excavated the corpses and the objects associated to them revealed other intricate details about the killings and the victims. The position of the bodies, laid down in pairs, superposed and adjusted to the man-made or *anthropic* shape of the dug-out terrain, suggested a type of premeditated planning and organization of the burial on the part of the perpetrators, to the archaeologist. Moreover, objects related to the abuse and assassination of these individuals made visible the aesthetics of their torture and death. Their forced disposition effected the brutality of their treatment as they appeared to be strongly tied by the wrists individually and to one another by the forearm, in pairs—with the exception of two corpses that were tied around their necks—with metal and cable wire. Multiple bullets and shells found in the bodies and in the surrounding area suggested these men had been executed in the vicinity of the burial ground (Muñoz Encinar 2011). Objects carried by each individual alluded to their personal habits, attire, or care, also suggesting that this unregistered group of eighteen men had been killed as they were being transferred elsewhere, possibly to another prison or detention site (ibid.).

In a similar way, Mass Grave 3 was found in what could have been the "*área de los desamparados*" or "zone of the helpless," where poverty-stricken neighbours would be buried, in particular, in the years of extreme famine that followed the conflict (Muñoz Encinar 2011). The remains, placed among other civil interments, coincided with some of the burials recorded in the cemetery registry book in 1943, according to the documentation compiled by Antonio López Rodriguez. Here, one of the entries designated "various irregular burials referred to as '*unknown*' and described as '*dead as a result of a clash with the Civil Guard*'" (ibid., 85; emphasis in original). In informal conversations during the excavation work, the archaeologists and Antonio López Rodriguez pondered the potential relation of these remains to a group of guerrilla fighters or *maquis* who might have been captured and later executed in the postwar years. Later, Antonio would further explore this hypothesis in the collective publication of the exhumation's results.[5] In his article, the data obtained from the corpses is related to that in the archival record and other historians' research, such as that of Benito Díaz Díaz (2011), who had documented a similar struggle between the Civil Guard and the guerrilla on the same date in Castuera.

The scientific scrutiny of the mass graves throughout the excavation turned these mortal remains and their significant objects into visible proof of violence, which gained, thereafter, different meanings in contact with activists' claims and familial experience. For some members of AMECADEC, these finds supported a desire to substantiate Francoist repression against other visions about the past. They reaffirmed the association's authority over the production of the history of the war in the locality, in a landscape of competing revisionist and political affirmations. Distinct members expressed these aspirations differently. For the families that often attended the exhumation, these finds intensified the individual memory of their kin and their wish to encounter them—as seen in the previous section—even if a positive identification seemed unlikely due to the poor preservation of the bones. In her study of the semiotic understandings of human remains in different scientific and social contexts, Zoe Crossland (2009) discusses the example of the body parts and skull of Australian nineteenth century bushranger Ned Kelly and the controversy over the meaning of his bones. She points out that the "bargaining [between scientific, social and familial claims] illustrates the way that [the] dead body moves seamlessly from being viewed as person to property to evidence" (Crossland 2009, 70).

As in Crossland and Abu El-Haj's studies, where archaeological and forensic remains are at the centre of profound political and cultural disputes, in Castuera, the unknown human remains of the mass graves often became vehicles for the reassertion of ideological positions. Throughout the exhumation, visits from different political representatives to the mass grave made the value of these corpses apparent in regional and local parties' agendas. Official appearances from politicians, such as the local PP town mayor, the regional leader from IU, or the national socialist delegate from PSOE, made patent the actuality of a PP–IU alliance at local level or the interest of a weakened regional Socialist Party in claiming the exhumation as part of their own historical memory project. Moreover, for many members of AMECADEC, who felt a common political purpose and shared historicity with the individuals buried in the grave, these corpses reaffirmed a common bond, as well as their role as a *political family* for these nameless bodies. This form of selective kinship was established upon a kind of ideological communion with the Republican killed and the sacrifice they made for their democratic ideas—as different members of the association explained to me. Mainly from third generations, some of these activists were profoundly moved by a need to follow and address a history they considered also their own (Feuchtwang 2011, 176).

Just as kinship metaphors become idiosyncratic of state nationalist discourses that craft imagined communities around land through ancestor-based alliances (see Verdery 1999; Anderson 1983; Yuval-Davis 1997), one could argue here that tracing a lineage with the war killed—sustained by learnt Republican histories and values—created a particular imagined community that actively demanded that these bodies form part of a particular genealogy. The perception of a shared past with the individuals in the mass grave instilled in some members of the association a sense of responsibility and obligation (Feuchtwang 2011, 175), but also a sense of entitlement over the investigation and the interpretation of the village's tragic past. These sentiments, which were often entangled with present ideological antagonisms and strivings, turned the corpses into clear forms of property that could be owned and protected from other interpretations and ideological projects. For instance, when on one occasion the previous socialist town mayor of Castuera visited the mass grave, accompanied by a reporter from the local press, he was asked to leave the site by some of the members of AMECADEC. Overwrought by ongoing dissension over the remembrance of the conflict in the village with the previous socialist group, some members of the association asked the PSOE leader to go, as the bodies, in their words, ***belonged*** to the association. "These bodies are our bodies!" screamed one of the activists, moved by a burgeoning tone of exasperation that manifested the tensions of a long battle between some members of the previous party and the association in the village.

This protective attitude toward the corpses found in Mass Graves 1 and 3 was also part of a contest over meaning involving not only different individual actors and left-wing groups but also revisionist voices in the village and the region at large. According to some members of the association and to Antonio, local revisionist arguments had long connected the dead in the mass graves at the rear of the cemetery with Republican soldiers killed at the nearby front. For historians like Antonio, this meant to deny the postwar violence exercised by the Franco regime. The results of the exhumation contradicted these assumptions in relation to the way the killings were perpetrated. In Mass Grave 1, for instance, the ballistic study of the site that Laura provides in her report shows how the men were shot with at least six different handguns (Muñoz Encinar 2011), in their heads (kill shots) as well as in the rest of their bodies. As Laura's hypothesis denotes, the weapons used, the profile of individuals in the grave, and the treatment of the bodies suggests that the group "might have been executed by a group from Falange" (ibid., 74), as executions by the military were often done with rifles—as seen in other exhumations. In Mass Grave 3, the archaeologist identifies a bullet in the ribcage of one of the corpses and the signs of antemortem violence on some of the skeletons. As stated above, the report concludes that, in relation to the documentation found, Civil Guards could have killed these men in 1943.

The case of the unknown human remains exhumed in the mass graves of Castuera triggered much uncertainty due to a lack of knowledge about their identities. For this reason, the final conclusions that Laura presents in her report were reached after many exchanges between archaeologists and historians, in which the data and references of the mass grave and the archive were constantly cross-examined. The contradiction and doubt that often conditioned the process of inferring an explanation about the mass graves were jointly negotiated through the superimposition of different sciences, which complemented each other's judgements (Latour 1999). Such exercises ultimately served to ascertain previous suppositions about the history of the Camp, which for many, could now further "disprove", as Guillermo León read in the manifesto, "those who assert that Francoist repression in *La Serena* never occurred". Moreover, uncertainty was also challenged by the appearance of material markers in the mass grave, which triggered other imaginings around the corpse, connecting these human remains to other possible identities and stories of disappearance.

Imagining Identity, Narrating Disappearance

In her study of DNA technology for the identification of Srebrenica's missing in Bosnia, Sarah Wagner (2008) has spoken about the role that material evidence plays in the articulation of scientific and familial accounts about a person's identity. In *To Know Where He Lies*, Wagner analyses how the objects and the possessions found with the human remains buried in primary and secondary mass graves associated with the massacre are treated within the space of the laboratory to extract as much information as possible, mainly from what the person wore and carried with them at the time of death. Objects such as jackets, trousers, or shoes, cigarette tins and holders, prayer beads, photographs, or books often facilitated the antemortem and the postmortem analysis of the expert. According to the forensic scientist with whom Wagner worked, these material remnants spoke about the life story of the individuals whilst living in the UN enclave prior to their flight and deaths, and provided clues about their identity and the way they died—sometimes showing whether they were tortured or how they were killed. Together with the antemortem information gathered from families, scientists make use of these objects in order to connect human remains with their relatives and to proceed to a final DNA identification.

Likewise, in Castuera, the emergence of an extensive variety of objects, especially in Mass Grave 1, had a decisive impact on the formulation of some scientific postulates during and after the exhumation. For instance, the numerous spoons that prisoners kept for their meals, or the coins, which confirmed the existence of an economy inside the detention site—as Antonio López has documented—hinted at the quotidian life within the Camp. Other items, of a more personal nature, pointed to the social pasts of these corpses, marking out the individual and group profiles of the bodies in the mass grave. Objects such as a crucifix found in the hand of one of the corpses (Fig 4.3) or the appearance of various religious medals suggested, for instance, as Muñoz pointed out in our interview, the person's confession or creed. In the case of the crucifix, when the archaeologist cleaned and restored the object, in the laboratory, she found an inscription on the cross ("*Jesus, José, Maria—Frentes y Hospitales*"), which revealed that these crucifixes had been produced by the female section of Falange. This led Antonio to consider whether the prisoner already had the crucifix, or whether it was given to the victim by a priest of the Francoist army that often confessed prisoners before their execution[6] (Laura Muñoz Encinar, Cáceres, 2011). Likewise, the religious medals found with some of the corpses gave clues about the area from which they might have originated, as particular Saints and Virgins evoked specific locations—as in the case of the medal of the Virgin of Guadalupe, the patron saint of Extremadura, and San Jerónimo, found with another corpse.

Other objects, such as a military insignia from the Republican Sanitary Personnel (*Cuerpo de Sanitarios de la República*) and another badge from the Railway Workers' Union (*Sindicato de Ferroviarios*) hinted clearly at the Republican identities of the victims (Muñoz Encinar 2013).

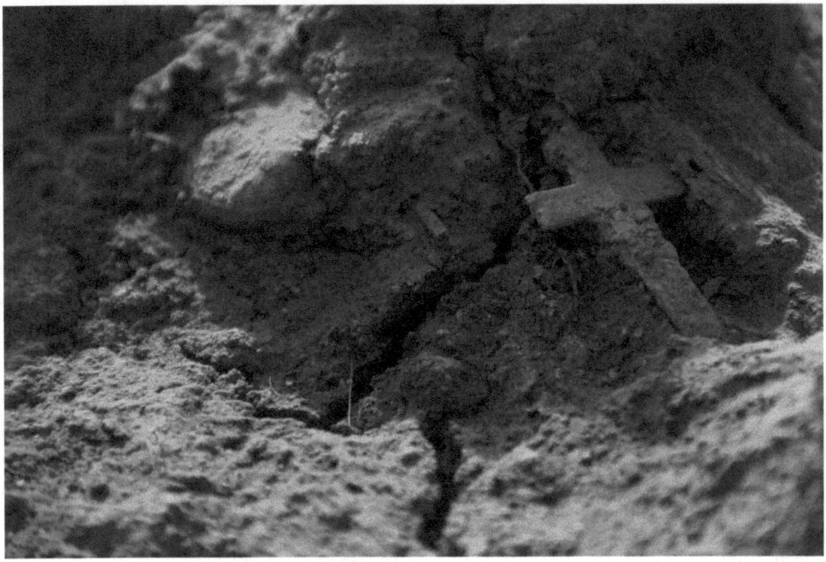

Fig. 4.3 Crucifix found in Mass Grave 1

These two objects pointed to the significant political roles of their owners, whom in both cases were found with multiple other possessions and traces of expensive garments, such as boots. This contrasted with the limited belongings that other corpses carried. Objects such as a pair of cufflinks or a wedding ring appeared next to other corpses, who only carried a pencil, a lighter, or a few coins. The different types of possessions that these corpses carried made Laura observe that the group was indeed a mixed group of men from different social backgrounds and occupations. Other enigmatic finds included two small pieces of paper, which remained nearly intact, according to the archaeologist, as they had been in contact with metal in the form of coins, cufflinks, and a cornet found with different bodies. When these were unearthed, one could not help but think of the fortuitous chemical reaction that had allowed them to persist in time, and allowed them to become pieces of distinguished importance for the archaeologist and the historian in the present for the writing they may contain.

Moreover, other objects also hinted at the familial and intimate affiliations of the deceased, as Renshaw (2011) has also observed in exhumations in northern Spain. For instance, the body of the man who belonged to the sanitary personnel of the Republican Army was found carrying a wallet that contained faded documentation. Later on, during her examination in the laboratory, Laura also encountered a lock of hair between the folds of the leather wallet. The perfectly preserved hair indicated, as the archaeologist would point out to me, an emotive personal relation with someone else—a child, a wife, a lover—inevitably evoking the image of rupture and a history of loss for the individual to whom it belonged. The appearance of the fragment of hair indeed inspired the hope of a possible identification for the team, as Antonio López Rodriguez had located a family whose relative was a doctor in the Republican army. Considering that the positive identification of all the bodies—whether through DNA matching or "classical markers of identity" in anthropological analysis (Rios et al. 2010, 27)—was burdened by their disparate origins, the absence of living relatives or the decayed condition of some key osseous parts, this find signified the possibility of ascertaining the name of at least one of the men, through the genetic information contained in the lock and that provided by a potential living relative—and beyond presumptive identification. For the researchers, this information was invaluable. Such a connection would finally relate the mass grave to a concrete life story, which may be entangled with the history of the Camp.

When Wagner (2008) speaks about the objects and belongings of Srebrenica's missing, she observes—evoking Hoskins' insights (1994)—how such materiality acted as a trigger or "prop" for the telling of a biographical memory for scientists and also relatives (see also Renshaw 2011). She acknowledges how the forensic scientist could only represent "the likenesses" of the victim "through photographs or narrative descriptions, so that [their] meanings may reveal themselves to the eyes and ears of the people who possess the intimate knowledge of the missing person" (Wagner 2008, 142). In contact with the gaze of family relatives, Wagner argues, these objects established a new connection between the memory of the victim and his or her death (ibid., 145). The belongings found with the human remains in Srebrenica's graves activated forms of storytelling about the life of the deceased. They also confirmed, the author remarks, the finality of their deaths for the family, for their materiality spoke explicitly about an intimate past, filled with shared experiences around these items: the trousers someone sewed for the deceased; the tobacco box the person made and that his living son immediately identified; the new wool socks the person wore before his flight. All of these prompted a form of recognition in the living that bones and skeletons could not provoke. These objects made the living remember, making memories the ultimate proof in substantiating scientific analysis and DNA testing (ibid.).

In contact with the families that often visited the site of the exhumations, in Castuera, the variety of objects encountered in Mass Grave 1 acquired the opposite effect, as these objects triggered the imagination and retelling of a personal experience of prolonged disappearance for families who might never find the corpse of their relative. The belongings of those in Mass Grave 1 mixed with families' histories of relentless search, which erupted in the exhumation arena seeking to fulfil a long-awaited individual consolation. During fieldwork in Castuera, I developed a constant relation with three families that often visited the site. These relatives were Ángel Sayabera, Aurora Navas Morillo, and Maria Hormeño and her daughter Marielo. In my conversations with them each talked about the unknown fate of their kin who had been killed in Castuera during the moment of the occupation in 1938 and at the end of the war in 1939. Their words often expressed how such disappearances marked a life of bewilderment and silence over the deaths of their ancestors. All three stories evoked the feelings of uncertainty they experienced over time due to the broken transmission of familial histories between those who survived the conflict and their offspring. Some of them, like Ángel or Aurora, were never told what happened to their kin. In the case of Maria, she remembers how, although her mother never spoke about it, her brothers and she realized what had happened to their father. "I never asked her because I knew it"—she once said to me in an interview. In Marielo's case, her grandfather's story was uttered intermittently, in parts, through her mother's accounts, and halted by the burden of transgenerational secrecy.

Information about the lives and deaths of their kin returned to these families through the searches into state archives that Antonio López Rodriguez had led for years, and through the investigation led by the families themselves, as in the case of Marielo's. As seen in Chap. 6, on many occasions these processes of document collection shed light on the relative's life during the war and before their death. They also revealed information about where and how they might have died. Searches in the archives aimed to fill in the blanks of these families' traumatic history and to reveal the inconclusive gaps that their disappearances had generated.

For some of these relatives, the absence of their kin marked an unsettled childhood and adult life. The incertitude over their kin's whereabouts and death triggered an inner urge to find them, to search for them in different places, and to see them again. Throughout their lives, this need had filled their everyday existence with ghostly visions of their ancestors, which intensified their desire to encounter them alive. Later, through the materiality of the grave in the context of the exhumation, these families hoped they could find the dead bodies of their relatives, to finalise a life-long search and alleviate their unresolved grief. The mass graves in Castuera cemetery entwined the story of these families with the presence of such orphan and unknown human remains, generating a wish to reencounter their kin among the nameless dead.

Ángel Sayabera's past was intimately embroiled with the history of the Camp and the local experience of war death. Before the war broke out, the Sayabera family had been widely known for their numerous garages and cinemas in the area, first in the neighbouring Campillo de Llerena and later in Castuera. Ángel's father was also a well-known figure and member of the Communist Party who wrote for news sources such as *Extremadura Roja* (Red Extremadura)—of which Ángel proudly preserved a copy to this day. In the mist of the war, the family split, causing his mother to stay with her youngest offspring in Castuera and his father to travel elsewhere with the eldest. This would be the last time Ángel saw his family, as he described to Laura and me in an interview. Testimonies from neighbours said that Ángel's mother was executed outside of the old cemetery in 1938. A handwritten placard that Ángel made and hung on the window of the cemetery commemorates the place of her execution. His father and brothers, captured after the war, went missing whilst in Castuera concentration camp in 1939. His third brother died whilst waiting to be given a reprieve for his sentence in the same year. Similar signs pay tribute to them in the space of the old detention site and at the rear of the cemetery. Eventually, Ángel went to live with his maternal grandparents, who brought him up together with some of his remaining siblings. Recalling the tense atmosphere in the house, he depicted the silence that his grandparents kept around the killings, perhaps, as he observed, in order to protect them. As he described, Ángel could imagine the family's tragic past through his grandmother's shattering crying. Nonetheless, the creeping uncertainty that surrounded these deaths launched Ángel into other searches during his adult life:

> When I was already married and living here [in the village of Llera], I thought my father had escaped (*estaba huído*) and had sought refuge in the mountains. I am telling you, I often wanted to put up a sign on the backside of my car that said: Ángel Sayabera. In case he turned up on a highway or a road, you know?" (Ángel Sayabera, Llera, 2011)

By attaching a sign with the name of his father to the back of the taxi he drove for decades around Spain, Ángel aimed to attract his attention in case he had survived imprisonment and hidden elsewhere in the countryside or the mountains—as many did after the war. Unlike his mother, his father's trail had been lost at the concentration Camp, from where he had sent a letter whilst in detention. The ambiguity around his death in stories and official files left a window open, such that Ángel could believe he was alive. Ángel's continuous search was an indirect product of the undisclosed character of his father's death and also his unknown burial place. In a similar manner, for Maria Hormeño and her daughter Marielo, details about the death of Maria's father, José Hormeño, remained hazy for years, as Maria was only five when he was taken away. The disappearance of Maria's father also remained unclear in the archive, which her daughter researched later on—see Chap. 6. As in the case of Ángel Sayabera, the disappearance of her father, however, haunted Maria throughout her childhood and later, during her adolescence in Barcelona.

Maria's father went to fight at the Republican front with his three brothers. During the occupation of 1938, Maria's family fled the village to seek refuge in other Republican territories. When the conflict ceased in 1939, her mother and one uncle met Maria's father and travelled back to Castuera. Maria remembered that after hearing Franco's message calling for people who had "no blood on their hands" to come back to their hometowns, the family decided to return. Maria described in hesitation and anger the moment of her father's disappearance: "When we arrived", she reminisced, "a man, I think it was a local policeman, took him away". According to the parts of the story that were passed on by Maria's mother to her daughter, after being captive in the village prison for some days, he was taken out (*lo sacaron*) and executed, presumably with a group of other prisoners. Her mother, she recalled, was never officially notified about her husband's death and instead found out through one of her neighbours. Her father's body was never searched for and its burial place is still unknown to this date. For the coming generations, details about his death were vague, as some things, according to Marielo, were "too painful" to be spoken about by members of the family. The perplexity and speculation about his whereabouts later on prompted in Maria, in her words, a "sickly" daily sentiment:

> Can you believe, that someone tells you when you are 13 or 14 years old that your father escaped and he is alive and he is living here and there? Then you become obsessed… And you are in a park and see people and you stare at them thinking: will he be one of these men? But I don't think he saved himself. When I went to Barcelona for the first time, I saw a man in the *Plaza Magistratura*—I think that was the name of the square —and I walked and looked at him, walked and looked at him. I thought it was my father and that he was going to recognize me and say something to me. You become obsessed. (Maria Hormeño, Castuera, 2011)

Speaking about the work of the "uncanny" in connection to the Argentinean *desaparecidos*, Ewa Domanska (2005) explains that much of what characterises the violent act of disappearance and its effects on those who survive, is precisely the ambiguity over the location and fate of the disappeared victim. In the Argentinean case, the acts of repression perpetrated by the government of the military junta of General Jorge Rafael Videla after the coup d'état of 1976 led to the detention, torture, and killing of thousands of citizens considered opposed to the regime in secret detention centres around the country. The bodies of the victims were often disposed of in places where they might never be found or burnt or battered so they could not be identified. In the aftermath of these killings and under a new government, families' positions—especially within the movement of the *Madres de la Plaza de Mayo*—diverged around the possibility of finding and exhuming the human remains of their relatives. Some wanted these corpses to be exhumed whereas others refused to acknowledge that the victims were dead in order to preserve their status as "disappeared". According to the latter position, this would avoid the crimes committed under the government of the junta to fall into oblivion. In this case, the act of disappearance, Domanska (ibid.) argues, situates the body of the missing in a liminal state between life and death, as a monstrous act, in a Freudian reading, which resists the reality of death but does not fully evade it. In similar manner, for the families in Castuera, disappearance became a permanent state, which placed the dead but also the living on a threshold in which mourning and justice became difficult to articulate throughout the years. Maria's fixation with the image of her father and her affliction was a reaction to this persistent and unexplained absence. Like Ángel, María saw the figure of her father wherever she went, as a spectre that never abandoned her or ceased to permeate her imagination.

Aurora Navas Morillo lost her mother when the war ended in 1939. Married to Antonio Navas Lora, a famous socialist leader in the town, Matilde Morillo spent the years of the war as a teacher in different villages of Extremadura and Castilla-La Mancha. There, she lived with her sisters, parents, and daughters whilst her husband fought in the front. When Daimiel, the town where Matilde lived, was occupied, she lost her job. After the battle of the *Bolsa de la Serena*, Antonio Navas knew that the war had been lost and proposed to Matilde to run away to a different country with their youngest daughter. Matilde's sisters encouraged her to do this and to later return to collect the rest of her children. At the last minute, as Aurora recalls from conversations she had later in her life with members of the family, she decided to stay behind with the rest of her relatives.

At the end of the war, Aurora's father, Antonio, left for the Spanish Levant to board a ship that would take him to Morocco, where he was detained in different labour Camps. Matilde, knowing she had not committed a crime, returned to Castuera with the rest of the family. Upon her arrival at the town's train station, Matilde was arrested and taken to the village prison. Aurora vividly recalls this moment, the noise of the station, the confusion of people and the military men and *falangistas* that waited at the platform, since she was already a toddler. According to Aurora, after this, Matilde was released on the condition that she gave declaration at the police station every day. One day, however, she knew she would not be back, for she gave her watch to her sister, for her daughters. In May 1939, Matilde was executed at the entrance of the village cemetery. After this, her body, Aurora recalled, would never be returned to the family or found:

> My cousin, who was 15 at the time, told me that two days [after the execution] she heard people say: 'last night they killed seven and one of them was Mr. Antonio Navas's wife.' Then, my cousin ran home and told my aunts. My cousin's father went to the authorities with his brother and his son to ask for the body of my mother back—we have always asked to have her body back, since the moment of her death. My uncle told them that

> she already had a niche in the cemetery and that they wanted to bury her in sacred ground because she was a Catholic. The authority turned around to him and told him: 'go away because you don't know what could happen to you if you keep asking for that'. My uncle told him: 'I don't know what else they could do to us!' [...] Then his brother looked at him, put his arm around his shoulder, and told him: 'let's go home because everything has already been decided here'. (Aurora Navas Morillo, Castuera, 2011)

The death of Aurora's mother, like that of Ángel's relatives or Maria's father, had remained unclear and unanswered since the moment it occurred, prompting her insecurity and hesitation around how and where it occurred. As Domanska points out in the Argentinian case, in the context of these open-ended searches, the body became the ultimate form of testimony on which the past could finally be inscribed and ascertained (2005, 403). It is this lack of a corpse and the scarce trace of the missing relative that also mark the experience of disappearance in Spain. In the context of the exhumation, the search for a relative among the unknown corpses in the mass grave was prompted by such unresolved uncertainty. Moreover, when these relatives visited the site of the exhumations in Mass Graves 1 and 3, it was not only the sight of the corpses that awakened the connection between the human remains and the misfortune of their own relatives. More powerfully, it was the personal objects, which Wagner (2008) observed could place unknown human remains into kinship and affiliative associations, which caused families to search for their kin's bodies at the burial sites.

Throughout the excavation, Marielo searched for the boots her grandfather wore at the time of his death among the varied footwear that appeared inside the mass grave, as if the object could finally certified the stories she had heard. The sight of the different military boots that were unearthed throughout the excavation prompted Marielo to remember her grandfather's attire, which her mother had often recalled for her in previous conversations. The boots triggered an inherited memory in Maria's daughter, which prompted her to imagine the corpse of her grandfather in the burial site. For Ángel, it was the presence of a pair of glasses, which he identified as those his father wore, that revived his search for the corpse of his relative. The glasses, which were found in the last days of the exhumation, were shown when the archaeologist presented the results of the excavation in Castuera, months after the work in the mass graves had concluded. In a similar way, when different pencils

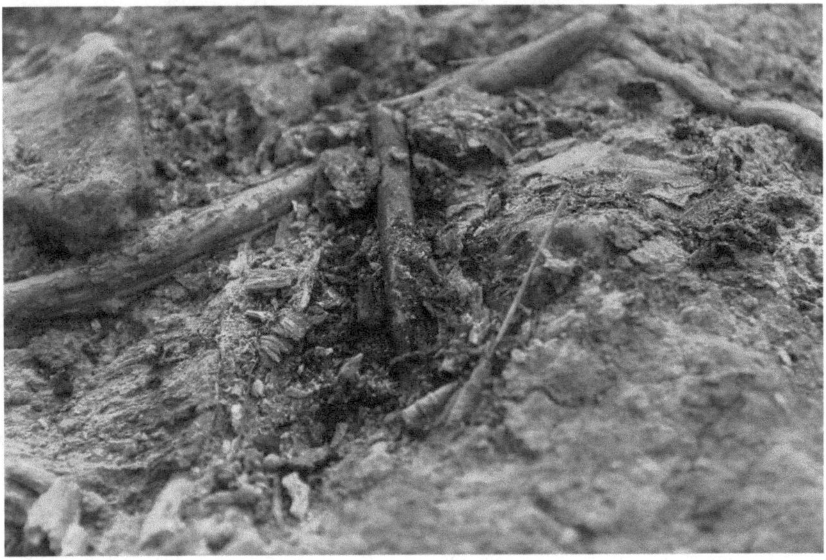

Fig. 4.4 Pencil found in Mass Grave 1

were unearthed in the excavation of Mass Grave 1, Aurora Navas Morillo enquired whether a woman had been found among the cadavers excavated by the team, as someone had told her that when her mother was killed she was tied to a painter who always carried pencils and paper with him. For her, these objects enlivened the prospect of a new search, as past attempts to locate her mother's grave led by PREMHEx in the same cemetery had proven unsuccessful (Fig. 4.4).

Families' willingness to reunite with the human remains of their missing kin thus mixed with the concreteness of the materials found, eliciting a renewed confidence in the search for their relatives. Such materiality was also, in the first place, the phenomenon that invoked these family's narratives about past suffering. Uttering these stories to archaeologists, volunteers, and historians in the public context of the exhumation was an attempt to inscribe the skeletons within a particular history of loss. Sarah Wagner (2008, 174) has argued, evoking Sartre, that in the absence of the body and of specific knowledge about a relative's death and whereabouts, imagination helps relatives to "take possession of the missing person's fate." In so doing, the objects of Mass Grave 1 also embodied the possibility of a positive identification, which could bring certainty to the family's quest and palliate their unresolved mourning through the scientific method. Indeed, the idea of a DNA match prompted hope for new explanations about the postmortem milieu of these families' missing. Confronted, however, with the vastness of the identification task in Castuera, some relatives understood the exhumation also as a space of "catharsis", as Maria's daughter, Marielo, explained to me towards the end of the exhumation. The excavation, as she stated, symbolized an event that allowed her to publically commemorate the memory of her grandfather.

In Castuera, the exhumation of the mass graves found inside the cemetery was conceived as a historical project to shed light over the functioning and existence of Castuera concentration camp and the repression in the area. The excavation of the unknown human remains found in Mass Graves 1 and 3 disclosed how the materiality of each burial site became evidence, which reasserted the legitimacy of the Camp's history and contested different historical and political visions in the present. The scientific interpretation of the corpses and their belongings mixed with the social, political, and familial worlds and anxieties that surrounded the exhumation. The archaeological and anthropological work performed at the mass grave and later on in the laboratory relied on historical information to deduce the ante-mortem story of the mortal remains. As the meanings of the materiality of the grave were negotiated between archaeologists, historians, activists, and families, different narratives started to take shape around the history of these men, their treatment and executions. The presence of such tangible evidence asserted the origin of the dead found in the mass grave. It prompted the telling of stories, which provided the human remains of the unknown with other subjective accounts and personal memories, and entangled the dead with the ghostly visions of the living. In the context of the exhumation, scientific evidence co-exists with intimate forms of memory work, placing individual life and death stories into collective understandings of the past.

Notes

1. According to the Ministry of Defence website, Ávila's Military Archive was created in 1993 due to the necessity of distributing the files held in the archives of the Terrestrial Army, in order to allow the latter to grow in the future. Ávila's Military Archive has held, since 1994, files related to the

Civil War (1936–1939), the Blue Division (sent to support the German government during World War Two), National Militia files, and information generated by the Ministry of the Army between 1939 and 1977 (see the Ministry of Defence website for more information http://www.defensa.gob.es/memoriahistorica/fuentes.html).

2. In an interview with Antonio López in 2011, the historian spoke about his work with different people that had collaborated with the institutions of the New Regime. His work with officials, such as one of the guards from the Camp, provided him with valuable insights into the daily routines within the detention site.
3. This is the trajectory that prisoners realized when they were transferred from the village prisons to the Camp.
4. A well-known priest and local historian of Francoist exploits, Angel David Martin Rubio, who is also the author of various books about the repression carried out by supporters of the Republican Popular Front (see Martín Rubio 2012), has vehemently argued for the remembrance of those who died fighting for the Francoist cause. A new blog, in which the historian collects a list of those killed by Republican forces or militia, advocates for the recovery of the names of the "heroes and martyrs" between 1936–1939.
5. The book, *De la ocultación de las fosas a las exhumaciones: la represión franquista en el entorno del Campo de Concentración de Castuera,* is a compilation of different articles containing the writings of historianswhich provided a sociopolitical context at time—archaeologists, and physical anthropologists that led the exhumations in 2011 and later in the second campaign realized in 2012. The collection was published and presented publically in the autumn of 2012.
6. In her report, Laura Muñoz Encinar specifies that, according to oral testimonies gathered by Antonio López Rodriguez from ex-prisoners from the Camp, detainees who were going to be killed were often allowed two concessions: to write a last letter to family members and to visit the priest before they died. According to Laura, Antonio López has also documented the existence of a priest in Catuera's Camp in Ávila's Military Archive (Muñoz Encinar 2011, 62).

References

Abu El-Haj, Nadia. 1998. Translating Truths: Nationalism, the Practice of Archeology and the Making of Past and Present in Contemporary Jerusalem. *American Ethnologist* 25 (2): 166–188.

Anderson, Benedict R. O'G. 1983. *Imagined Communities: Reflections on the Origin and Spread of Nationalism*. London: Verso.

Crossland, Zoë. 2009. Of Clues and Signs: The Dead Body and Its Evidential Traces. *American Anthropologist* 111 (1): 69–80.

Daston, Lorraine, and Elizabeth Lunbeck. 2011. *Histories of Scientific Observation*. Chicago: University of Chicago Press.

Díaz Díaz, Benito. 2011. La represión franquista como generadora del fenómeno de los huidos en Extremadura. *Revista de Estudios Extremeños* 67 (2): 909–933.

Ewa Domanska. 2005. Toward the Archaeontology of the dead body. *Rethinking History* 9 (4): 389–413.

Ferrándiz, Francisco. 2011. Autopsia social de un subtierro. *Isegoría: Revista de Filosofía Moral y Política* (45): 525–544.

Feuchtwang, Stephan. 2011. *After the Event: The Transmission of Grievous Loss in Germany, China and Taiwan*. New York: Berghahn Books.

Foucault, Michel, and Colin Gordon. 1980. *Power/Knowledge: Selected Interviews and Other Writings, 1972/1977*. Brighton: Harvester Press.

González, José Ramón. 2006. Prisioneros del miedo y control social: El campo de concentración de Castuera. *Hispania Nova. Revista de Historia Contemporánea*, 6.

Hacking, Ian. 1996. Memory Sciences, Memory Politics. In *Tense Past: Cultural Essays in Trauma and Memory*, ed. Michael Lambek and Paul Antze. London: Routledge.

Hinojosa Durán, José. 2009. *Tropas en un frente olvidado: El ejército republicano en Extremadura durante la Guerra Civil*. Editora Regional de Extremadura. Extremadura: Agapea.

Koselleck, Reinhart. 2004. *Futures Past: On the Semantics of Historical Time*. New York: Columbia University Press.

Lambek, Michael and Paul Antze. 1996. Introduction: Forecasting Memory. In *Tense Past: Cultural Essays in Trauma and Memory*, ed. Michael Lambek and Paul Antze. London: Routledge.

Latour, Bruno. 1999. *Pandora's Hope: Essays on the Reality of Science Studies*. Cambridge, MA and London: Harvard University Press.

León Cáceres, Guillermo, Antonio D. López Rodriguez, and José Ramón González Cortés. 2011. El campo de concentración de Castuera: del olvido forzado a lugar de memoria y recurso didáctico. *Revista de Estudios Extremeños* 67 (2): 527–594.

López Rodríguez, Antonio D. 2006. *Cruz, bandera y Caudillo: el campo de concentración de Castuera*. La Serena: CEDER.

López Rodriguez, Antonio D. 2013. La configuración de la memoria franquista en La Serena (1939–1948): materialies para su estudio. *La represión franquista en el entorno del Campo de Concentración de Castuera*, ed. Laura Muñoz Encinar, Xurxo M. Ayán Vila. and Antonio D. López Rodriguez.

AMECADEC, Spanish Ministry of the Presidency and CSIC-INCIPIT, pp.13–28.

Martín Rubio, Ángel D. 2012. *Extremadura: de la República a la España de Franco*. Madrid: Ediciones Barbarroja.

Meskell, Lynn. 2002. Negative Heritage and Past Mastering in Archeology. *Anthropological Quarterly* 75 (3): 557–574.

Muñoz Encinar, Laura. 2011. Memoria arqueológica de la excavación y exhumación de 2 fosas comunes del Franquismo localizadas en el cementerio de Castuera (Badajoz) INT/2011/102. Extremadura: University of Extremadura.

Muñoz Encinar, Laura. 2013. Exhumación en el cementerio de Castuera. Campaña 2011. In *De la ocultación de las fosas a las exhumaciones. La represión franquista en el entorno del Campo de Concentración de Castuera*, ed. Laura Muñoz Encinar, Xurxo M. Ayán Vila, and Antonio D. López Rodriguez. Extremadura: AMECADEC, Ministerio de la Presidencia de España and CSIC-INCIPIT, pp. 62–115.

Renshaw, Layla. 2011. *Exhuming Loss: Memory, Materiality and Mass Graves of the Spanish Civil War*. Walnut Creek, CA: Left Coast.

Ríos, Luis, José Ignacio Casado Ovejero, and Jorge Puente Prieto. 2010. Indentification Process in the Mass Graves from the Spanish Civil War. *Forensic Science International* 199 (1–3): e27–e36.

Verdery, Katherine. 1999. *The Political Lives of Dead Bodies: Reburial and Postsocialist Change, The Harriman Lectures*. New York: Columbia University Press.

Vila Izquierdo, Justo. 1999. *La Guerra Civil en Extremadura*. Badajoz: Universitas Editorial.

Wagner, Sarah E. 2008. *To Know Where He Lies: DNA Technology and the Search for Srebrenica's Missing*. Berkeley: University of California Press.

Young, Craig, and Duncan Light. 2012. Corpses, Dead Body Politics and Agency in Human Geography: Following the Corpse of Dr Petru Goza. *Transactions of the Institute of British Geographers* 38 (1): 135–148.

Yuval-Davis, Nira. 1997. *Gender & Nation*. London: Sage.

CHAPTER 5

Exhuming Familial Remains

A year after the exhumation in Castuera, in the summer of 2012, I joined Laura Muñoz Encinar's team in the excavation carried out in the village of Puebla de Alcocer. Contrary to the case in Castuera, the corpses searched for in the vicinity of Puebla—as people often referred to the village—belonged to a group of neighbours killed in an episode of postwar violence. Just like the unknown bodies found in Castuera, the men found in the mass graves of Puebla de Alcocer had been executed at the wake of the conflict in 1939. Nonetheless, their identities were not remote but well known to those in the village community. The memory of the people buried in these mass burial sites was ultimately part of the entangled histories of young and older generations. Their presence had never ceased to exist in the family and even communal repertoire of stories, which imagined the tragic experiences of some of its neighbours whilst mapping distinct kin affiliations and political relations. Marking a landmark in the community's history, some of the relatives, and especially the elders who were still alive at the time of the exhumation, had always known these men's fate and burial place and could remember the events of their detention and execution.

Promoted by a group of families from Puebla, the exhumation was still part of PREMHEx investigative efforts to examine the repressive modes of Francoist violence. It also, however, aimed to recover the remains of the ancestors of members of the locality to place them in the village's cemetery, with other community dead, in an attempt to restore

Z. Aragüete-Toribio, *Producing History in Spanish Civil War Exhumations*, World Histories of Crime, Culture and Violence,
DOI 10.1007/978-3-319-61270-6_5

their identity as kin but also as once-members of Puebla's public life. From the beginning, the exhumation was supported by the ruling local socialist administration, which envisioned the exhumation as a restorative act for the collective memory of the village. This bond shared with the corpses shaped the character of the exhumation project as well as the scientific analysis of the mass graves. The knowledge of the killings, which had been passed on between generations, was definitive in the making of the historical event that the archaeological analysis of the mass graves produced. Scientific evidence, in this case, was negotiated with the certainty of stories about the executions and the identities of those who were found in the grave. Here, relatives had the certainty of how and where their relatives had died. Hence, people often spoken of the executions, evoking less frequently, the notion of disappearance that other accounts of extrajudicial terror had generated in Castuera.

This chapter focuses on the way scientific practice interacted with the social and familial memory of the killings that existed in the village. In so doing, it pays special attention to the way kin transmission and social storytelling engaged with the identification of the dead in order to foreground their place in the community's collective memory. The chapter continues by discussing a concern with the way in which scientific objects trigger familial retellings of the past, which was introduced at the end of the previous case study of Castuera. Considering—as other anthropological works have done (Cruikshank 1998, 2005; Filippucci 2010; Pine 2007; Bloch 1996; Boyarin 1994; Feuchtwang 2011)—how oral histories enable particular forms of being-in-history across generations, the chapter explores how established kin and community memories about the killings are contested, complemented, and informed by scientific bearings. Ultimately, my aim is to discuss how these social stories, which often overshadowed scientific evidence, ascertained connections between descendants and the missing and validated a biological bond that could not be restored by scientific analysis.

The Search for the Village's Mass Graves

In 2011, José Sánchez-Paniagua Bayón initiated the search for the body of his grandfather, who had been killed and buried with other neighbours in the cavities of two trenches situated today in two privately own plots a few kilometres outside of Puebla de Alcocer, in the middle of the countryside. According to José, the wish to learn about the whereabouts of his relative's corpse and the possibility of recovering it had always intrigued him and been present in his thoughts "as far back as [he] could remember" (José Sánchez-Paniagua, Puebla, 2012). José, however, had also collaborated in the search for other victims of postwar violence. In 2006, José participated in the exhumation of the body of his wife's uncle, a guerrilla fighter killed by the Civil Guard and buried in a village in the province of Cuenca (Castilla-La Mancha) on his return from exile in France in the 1940s. Later on, he carried on cooperating with the historical memory association in Cuenca (ARMH Cuenca), who had enabled the previous excavation, in the investigation of other cases and the exhumation of other human remains.

Taking part in these initiatives incited José to actively start the process of recovering his grandfather's remains "and those of his neighbours" (José Sánchez-Paniagua, Puebla, 2012), motivated by a personal urge to comply with what he saw as "an act of justice" (ibid.). José's father, also called José, who was, back in 2012, nearly 84 years old, had also long hoped for the reburial of his father's remains in the village cemetery. With newly found motivation and energy from the two previous exhumations, José set out to research the history of the executions, their traces in village elder's memories, and in the municipal archive, whose files contained dispersed information about the repression perpetrated by ruling postwar political elites in 1939. After compiling information about the other men in the mass grave, he tried to contact their families—although he admits that it was impossible to find all of them, as some had disappeared and others did not want to get involved in the exhumation. With support from those willing to collaborate, he created the Association of Families of Victims of [Francoist] Repression in Puebla de Alcocer and later applied for an exhumation grant from the Ministry of the Presidency, approved before the general elections of November 2011.

When we first met, in June 2012, José told me that the fundraising process had been arduous, as I had already heard from other people in PREMHEx and AMECADEC, though not as complex and bewildering, it seemed, as the process of requesting permits to excavate the mass graves from the Heritage Office. As also happened in Castuera, the delayed release of an official permit to excavate from the regional government caused the association and also José much consternation. José's worry was the matter of time. We met five months after José had applied for the permit. At this time, additional documentation was still being requested from the association. José appeared frustrated by the ongoing demands for further information and reiterated the need to speed up these proceedings, as some older relatives were already passing away. The widow and daughter of two of the men in the mass graves had died in the months prior to our interview. José's resentment became especially evident as he used the space of our interview, recorded in audio and video format, to denounce the situation. He hoped I could give him an answer, but I had none. By that time, pressure, however, was already being exerted on the Heritage Office in 2012—especially by PREMHEx—to create a special clause in the law that dealt with the specificities of mass grave exhumations.

In contrast to this deceptive experience with the regional administration, at a local level, the active backing of the socialist town hall heavily influenced the context in which the exhumation in Puebla de Alcocer unfolded. In a small village where public opinion had always been marked by the tensions between left- and right-wing views and the polarised agendas of the two political forces, PP and PSOE, endorsing the recovery of these bodies was a political move in line with the socialist historical memory programme that enjoyed the approval of some and provoked the unease and rejection of others. The town mayor assured me that the exhumation project was a contested issue among neighbours and political representatives. According to him, the historical memory propositions of PSOE had always been met with the dismissal of PP city councillors in the village. He pointed out in an informal conversation that they had "always found [themselves] alone in relation to the matter". Nonetheless, ultimately, their majority government allowed for the development of contended projects such as the exhumation of Puebla's Republican dead.

On the other hand, as a member of the regional parliament, the mayor was also critical of the role of the Heritage Office in the administration of permits for Civil War-related excavations. According to him—and as many directly involved in associations also observed after the general election—these projects had been intentionally drawn out and slowed down by an uninterested conservative ruling party. One has to acknowledge, however, that the activity of the Heritage Office was also slow when PSOE occupied the regional government—as proven in Castuera case—however, bureaucratic processes worsened as a result of PP's unwillingness to address activities connected to the memory of the Civil War and postwar violence. The town mayor and Member of Parliament ascertained that left-wing parties like his or IU should also press the current government on the patrimony issue—something that is not often done, if at all (Manuel Moreno Delgado, Puebla, 2012). In the village, he noted, these adverse positions could also be strongly felt. In the framework of these disparate ideological positions in regional and local settings, his was clearly a politically-motivated contribution. Nonetheless, it was accompanied by a desire to bring neighbours closer, for he envisioned the exhumation as an act that could "repair" the community's social fabric. As he anticipated before the exhumation started:

> One of the problems we will have to deal with is the issue that some people will try—and José knows this—to argue that there are more important things to do right now, that this is not necessary, that where are we going with this… and people would make these comments with those who have their loved ones buried where they should be, in the cemetery, with their commemoration and things… The rest of people don't have them. We cannot forget that they are neighbours from the village and I, as representative of the Institution have the obligation to simply correct that anomaly in the municipality. That anomaly has to be corrected. Neighbours have to be buried in the municipal cemetery, following any ritual, but in the municipal cemetery. I am not going to allow any meddling of that kind from people that might feel now annoyed or uncomfortable… We must do what we really ought to do and what relatives want to do with their loved ones and I think no one can argue with that—and of course, we must do it also at an institutional level […] This is an anomaly, which one might think doesn't exist because people don't speak about it, but it does exist and it needs to be dealt with as soon as possible—at least to give the most direct relatives of those executed, of those repressed, the satisfaction of fulfilling that hope: 'I can take flowers or I can remember my father and brothers or whoever, whenever', and this is what we are going to do. (Manuel Moreno Delgado, Puebla, 2012)

The town mayor's words subtly evoke the strained relation between different members of the community and make visible the institutional commitment that would, later on, during the exhumation, affect the type of historical and memory work performed in relation to the killings. As the mayor, José, and other neighbours shared with me on multiple occasions, much of the animosity between right- and left-wing village families was still marked by issues rooted in the war past, especially among the older generations who had experienced the conflict directly or indirectly. The social struggle around property and class inequality influenced political standpoints before and during the war and caused many of the violent episodes people would later describe to me. After the war, as Manuel, the town mayor, clarified, these disparities increased, especially as the poverty-stricken families of the defeated were subordinated to the "fear and injustice" (ibid.) of the new local Francoist authorities and their collaborators.[1] Though these confrontations were not as pronounced in the present, some say divisions lasted until the 1990s.

Some also commented that prior to the exhumation, a group of neighbours had attempted to boycott an informative event about the exhumation that took place in the village in 2011. This bitterness then, was still present in Puebla's public realm. The perseverant tone of the mayor's words and his will to "correct" what he sees as an "anomaly" should be understood in the framework of such an ongoing social friction. Fear but also disconformity led many, according to the town mayor, to assert that the dead "should not be touched" and "should be left where they are" (ibid.). Younger generations however, according to Manuel, seemed to have a more forward-looking approach to the unearthing and reburial of these corpses. In our first interview, the mayor made a point about the one-sidedness of past commemorative efforts and the resolute reburial and tributes that the right-wing dead had enjoyed throughout the dictatorship. In this light, the mayor implied, the exhumation of the defeated would mend an unbalanced situation and thus, in his words, "advance freedom and a normal coexistence" between neighbours in the twenty first century (ibid.). Thus, for the socialist leader, providing these bodies with a "proper burial" in the municipal cemetery would effectively influence social rapport within the community. According to José, in the context of the village politics, promoting the history of these executions would have been gruelling under a PP government. The impetus given to the search for the bodies in 2011 contrasted with a previous attempt to find the mass graves in 1992. As happened in other villages, back in the 1990s, the then PSOE town mayor sought to collect the signatures of villagers in support of the excavation, in an effort to rally the support of the whole community; however, as José and Manuel explained, "there was still too much fear" among villagers and the initiative never prospered.

In Puebla, the town hall facilitated access to research sources and logistical aspects of the location and excavation campaigns, and made some neighbours more receptive and tolerant towards the initiative. The town hall's support allowed José to make extensive and in-depth investigation into the files contained in the municipal archive. There, he studied the civil registry and the death certificates issued in 1939 and compiled two lists with the names of the men who had died that year, and whose cause of death read "*dead as result of a clash with the public force*". Additionally, he was also able to draw on other documentation that displayed the workings of governmental surveillance, the management of suspects, and the administration of prison sentences locally. The archive offered clues that allowed José to piece some parts of the story of the executions together; however, its scattered abundance and the fact that some files—such as those that belonged to the time of the Second Republic—had been burned and destroyed when the war ended, made the information vague and the use of other versions of the story necessary.

In relation to the executions, the civil registry provided José with the names and surnames of the victims and situated the events on two exact days. The first group was executed on the 21st May 1939, whilst the second was taken out on the 25th May 1939. The death certificates of these men was the only information contained in the municipal records about the killings (see the death certificate of José's grandfather in Fig. 5.1). As José observed in one of our interviews, these men, thirty-seven according to the archive, were "detained, imprisoned and killed", but there was no trail of such punishment, no court-martial or additional procedures that might have generated other types of data about their deaths. For José, the lack of other documents—for instance, from a court-martial—exemplified the lack of a fair trial these men had faced, and hence the impossibility of defending their lives before a court of law. The archive disclosed the identification of those killed, but it did not reveal the space of their burial or details about how the killings took place. The absence of other documentation, such as sentences or court summaries, buttressed the furtive nature of these deaths, accentuating their incomprehensibility for families.

Compiling information about the killings in Puebla opened a window on the tragic past of the village, but also displayed the trails of a "social history of remembering" (Burke 1989, 100; Jing 1996) that revealed the difficulties and hazards of transgenerational transmission. José's archival research was paired with an investigation into personal accounts connected to the event of the killings. It was through the memories that some neighbours still had about the executions that José was able to locate the mass grave. Since childhood, José remembered, his father had told him and his sister Consuelo (also part of the families' association) "more or less" where the bodies were buried. Although José's widowed

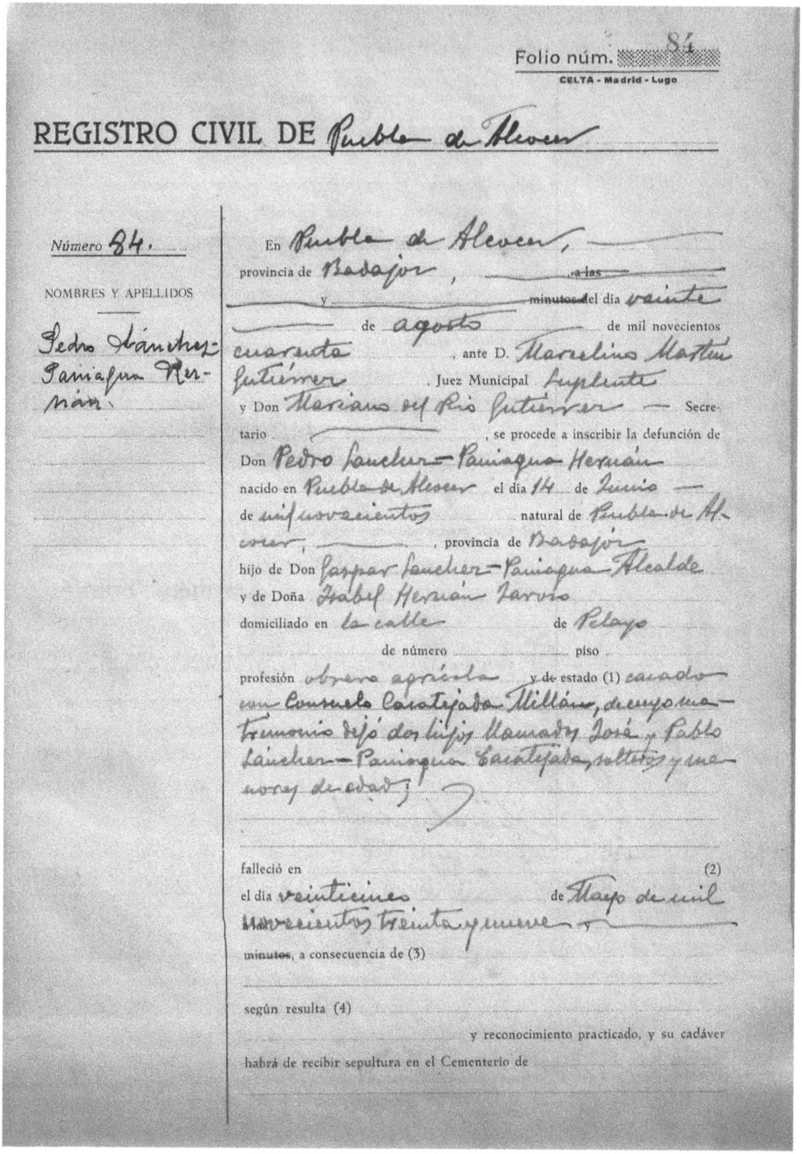

Folio núm. 84

CELTA - Madrid - Lugo

REGISTRO CIVIL DE Puebla de Alcocer

Número 84.

NOMBRES Y APELLIDOS

Pedro Sánchez-Paniagua Hernán.

En Puebla de Alcocer, provincia de Badajoz, a las y minutos del día veinte de agosto de mil novecientos cuarenta, ante D. Marcelino Martín Gutiérrez, Juez Municipal suplente y Don Mariano del Río Gutiérrez — Secretario, se procede a inscribir la defunción de Don Pedro Sánchez-Paniagua Hernán nacido en Puebla de Alcocer el día 14 de Junio de mil novecientos natural de Puebla de Alcocer, provincia de Badajoz, hijo de Don Gaspar Sánchez-Paniagua Alcalde y de Doña Isabel Hernán Barrios domiciliado en la calle de Pelayo de número piso profesión obrero agrícola y de estado (1) casado con Consuelo Caratejada Millán, de cuyo matrimonio dejó dos hijos llamados José y Pablo Sánchez-Paniagua Caratejada, solteros y menores de edad;

falleció en (2) el día veinticinco de Mayo de mil novecientos treinta y nueve y minutos, a consecuencia de (3)

según resulta (4) y reconocimiento practicado, y su cadáver habrá de recibir sepultura en el Cementerio de

Fig. 5.1 Death certificate of Pedro Sánchez-Paniagua. Courtesy of José Sánchez-Paniagua

grandmother had never shared explicit details about her husband's murder with her son or grandchildren—according to José, to protect them from potential reprisals—members of the family had always had a general idea about their relative's death and burial place in Puebla's countryside. Other village elders seemed to have more accurate knowledge about the location of the mass grave, which helped José to contrast his father's insights on the whereabouts of the mass internments and expand on the information held in archival documents. Even if many people did not openly talk about these repressive episodes of the end of the conflict, the image of the mass graves had always been present in the collective memory of the village.

According to José and Consuelo, many older people knew where the bodies were because their own parents had told them about the executions or they had worked in the surrounding areas of the mass grave for years. The fact that dead men in the two trenches from the war had been left exposed for some days after being killed and later lightly buried until 1952—when the terrain was partitioned and their new owners fully covered them to cultivate the land—left many with vivid recollections of the shootings and of the presence of the decomposing bodies in the middle of the fields. José also spoke to some of those who had experienced the events originally, like the men's widows and offspring still alive before the exhumation. The memories of some of these women were especially poignant, for a few of them had secretly, some days after the executions, tried to cover the bare bodies with the little soil they could gather using small wicker baskets they carried with them. Among these women was José and Consuelo's grandmother. One of them, alive at the time of the search, had told José what she remembered about that day, providing him with additional information about the area where the bodies lied. When he began the process of locating the mass graves, José relied on the testimony of these older interlocutors and, taking his father, other elder neighbours of Puebla and the renting owners of the plots to the large estate, he set the search for the bodies in motion:

> I took my father and four other elders—among them, the plots' owners. They took me to the place and told me: "here they are". They even told me stories—though they were very young back then—about what their parents told them in relation to the men executed, to where they were […]. For instance, the owner of the plot where my grandfather is buried told us that he used to go there to plough with his father, to grow cereals

> (oats, wheat, barley...) and every time they went over the area where the trench is located his father would tell him: "let's not plough too deep here because we might pull something out, we might find something". Stories like these... (José Sánchez-Paniagua, Puebla, 2012)

The grave was thus found through the information these neighbours provided to José, as no other document existed about the place of the killings. As happened in Castuera, personal experiences connected to the mass graves facilitated the location work and became an intrinsic part of the archaeological process. In her study of the Podhale in Poland, Frances Pine (2007) has argued how intimate memories entrenched in everyday spaces and features of the landscape can become props for the remembrance of bigger events that affected individual and familial experience over time. In Puebla, ***knowing*** about the killings became, for many, commonplace, entangled with quotidian village life—especially as many work (e.g., farming, cattle raising) and leisure activities (e.g., hunting) still happen today in the area where the executions took place. During my time in Puebla, and as I spoke to people before and during the exhumation, other stories and rumours about the presence of the graves and bodies in people's everyday memory elucidated their lingering impression in the community's imagination. Some retold, on occasions, the way in which other neighbours had found dogs carrying body parts back from the mass graves—some stories spoke of a hand, others of a leg—just outside the village. Many of these stories spoke of the gruesome reality of the killings through these uncanny encounters, evoking the mass graves' afterlife in the postwar village and the active countryside milieu. At this early stage, when José took these neighbours to the site where the executions occurred, testimonies delineated the excavation ground.

These contrasted with other stories—such as one told by the main landowner of the large estate where the trenches were located—who denied the bodies were there until the moment the mass grave was opened. According to José, before the archaeological prospection of the land was undertaken, with the help of members from PREMHEx such as Cayetano Ibarra, they also used ground-penetrating radar, broadly used in localisation endeavours of human remains in Spain. As José told me, this tool helped them to be "sure" of the location. The radar, which scans the soil, producing an image of the terrain underground with its changes in materials and structure, provided, in José's words, "a positive report", as it identified the same area that testimonies had singled out.[2] The technological device seemed to offer a form of validation and certainty for the family and some project members. As in Castuera, the presence of scientific technologies and performance comingled with personal accounts of the past, transforming people's imagination about the executions. As the materiality of the mass graves was uncovered, these stories gained a profuse and expansive character, drawing a portrait of postwar suffering and further repression in the village.

Assembling a History of the Executions

The event of the executions in Puebla had a profound impact on many neighbours' lives, as it affected numerous left-wing—mainly socialist—families in the village. The executions had been subtly recalled in family circles and so their memory had been passed on from those who experienced the event firsthand to later generations of kin and close neighbours. When the exhumation started in July 2012, the mass gravesite was filled with the voices of those who lived through the end of the conflict and remembered it vividly, and the vicarious memories of younger members of the community—neighbours, children, and grandchildren of the people who lay in the mass burial site. The exhumation also attracted visits from people from neighbouring villages, who had heard about the unearthing of the bones. It also awakened the interest of members of the Civil Guard and the judicial police, who filed a report about the bodies found—something Laura had rarely seen in other exhumations, as she would later observe. At the mass grave, people recounted their version of the story of the killings personally to me or as part of small group conversations that formed next to the archaeological dig. In such retellings, one could appreciate the contrasting and similar aspects they all contained. These oral narratives were conditioned by the way in which events had been lived or learnt, by singular anecdotal additions and people's particular interpretations. Nonetheless, they all seemed to share common details about the detention, execution, and burial of these men.

According to many of these stories, most of the men, of socialist ideology and affiliation, were arrested and imprisoned in the spring of 1939, when Francoist troops entered the locality and ended with the Republican government that ruled the village until the end of the war. After being held in the old prison, situated in what is today the elders' bar (*hogar del pensionista*), they were moved to a convent that had been turned into a prison, located at the edge of the village—appropriated during the war for military purposes by Republicans and later, at the end of the contest, by Francoist troops. Whereas some stories mentioned the prison and convent, others never addressed it. Many family members that spoke to us during the exhumation asserted that their relatives had never been jailed and instead had been taken straight from their houses for execution. Older members of the community remembered that the weather was already warm when the first group of men were put on a truck and driven to the area of *Cuesta de la Cabeza*, one of the plots where the first trench was located. Days later, two other trucks were filled with the remaining men, so the story goes, and transported to another area, known today by the name of *El Chaparral*. Both plots are today part of a large estate called *Bodegones*, located near an area commonly known as *El Morro*, a point of reference for many in the local community. According to some stories, the men were summoned and driven to the two sites by Francoist military and right-wing neighbours from Puebla. After the men were killed—some stated that as soldiers refused to do it, two young men from the village were placed in charge of carrying out the shootings—the bodies were left exposed and guarded for a few days, until some of the widows managed to evade the appointed military controls on a point known as *Aldeavieja*, in the outskirts of the village, in order to cover them with some soil.

At the exhumation site, these stories filled the space, as the team excavated the two trenches, situated within the field of holm oak trees, olive trees, and brooms of *Bodegones*. These accounts, which some uttered and some heard from fellow neighbours for the first time, were made common, unravelling distinct renderings of the executions garnered through familial exchanges over time and forming a collective perception of the events. At the mass grave, communal sharing of first- and second-generation accounts, influenced by a history of secretive storytelling and also rumour, attempted to piece together an image of what *really* happened in the past, creating a "shared sense of being-in-time" (Pickering and Keightley 2013, 121) or a "sense of living connection" (Hirsch 2008, 104). As the town filled with families returning for the summer *fiesta* at the time of the excavation, these individual and familial stories entered the public realm, in an act of conscious recollection, becoming incorporated into the village's social memory. Testimonies and conversations were primarily shared at the exhumation site, though they also penetrated people's interactions in the village scene.[3] At the mass grave, discussions and impressions among neighbours such as José, his sister Consuelo, and other visitors, wrestled with a history that could not be fully grasped, seeking coherence in the certainty and uncertainty contained in these lived and borrowed oral accounts. The difficulties in the transmission of some of these memories, often encrypted by the experience of individual suffering of a previous generation, especially in the postwar years, marked the speculative character of some of these narratives during the exhumation. Established versions of the events mixed with moments of hesitance where gaps in people's knowledge of the killings motivated the ongoing work of the collective imagination. During fieldwork, I became interested in the nature of these at-times fragmented and blurred accounts, and especially in the ways in which people aimed to conjointly resolve these cracks, through the untangling of incoherent clues found within the stories, the archive, and in connection to the findings of the archaeological team in the mass grave.

In such a way, unmediated and mediated narratives about the tragic event coexisted throughout the exhumation, elucidating the way in which intergenerational acts of transfer occurred within families and neighbours and intra-generational encounters happened among members of second generations (Pickering and Keightley 2013). The formulation of these oral accounts within the group setting displayed, on the one hand, forms of recall attached to a lived past by elders who gave testimony of what they saw when they were younger. On the other, there were inherited memories acquired from elders' life histories—whether relatives or neighbours—by the children and grandchildren of the defeated, which, as Marianne Hirsch (2008, 107) has observed when describing the concept of *postmemory*, are "not mediated by recall but by imaginative investment, projection and creation." Other families however, were inevitably distrustful in sharing their family's past and often guarded their stories, as they feared that the exhumation and the telling of some stories might "awake the revenge of others". In such a way, the story of the killings was assembled through exchanges across generations and between members of the same age groups, articulating the village collective mnemonic imagination (Pickering and Keightley 2013)—formed by heterogeneous views about the past and how it should be articulated.

Moreover, these perceptions and experiences of the past also differed in terms of their ideological standpoint, since not all socialist neighbours and families that attended the exhumation shared the same versions and these manifold visions were also constructed in relation to the views of right-wing neighbours who, on occasions, also visited the gravesite. The memory of the killings was, in the words of Michael Rothberg (2009, 3), multidirectional and "subject to ongoing negotiation, cross-referencing, and borrowing" between those who came into contact through the exhumation. The assemblage of a historical memory of the executions was a dialogical and dialectic exercise between the members of the community and the material objects found, such as human remains or documents. These encounters often revealed tensions, which emerged when distinct portrayals of the past were brought into contact with one another. They adverted the idiosyncrasies of a social identity engendered through years of conflict but also through coexistence between neighbours.

When the team began to excavate the first trench in the area of *El Chaparral* (named TR1 in the archaeological record), the first human and material traces that appeared within the zigzagging trench disconcerted scientists and villagers alike. As mentioned above, according to elders' stories, two trucks took a group of men who were killed and buried together inside the trench. This is the story that second and third generations like José's learnt and retold until the day the mass grave was unearthed. The list of names that José compiled from the municipal archive, which suggested the apparent split and execution of these men into two different groups and days, consolidated the belief that the bodies of twenty-six men were buried in the first trench whilst the human remains of twelve other individuals had been inhumed in the second, located in *Cuesta de la Cabeza*. This seemed highly likely for those such as José and his family, closely involved in the historical research process and thus aware of such archival information. The appearance of only eight corpses in the first excavated area of the trench filled families, and particularly José, with a deep sense of incredulity and mistrust when they approached the mass grave.

As the team worked to expose the bones and their belongings, José and other visitors discussed where the rest of the bodies might be. Doubts concerning the possibility of finding all the corpses started to emerge, causing a palpable sense of unease among families. From the beginning, and as the inside of the mass grave was hollowed, Laura Muñoz Encinar prudently shared with me her own qualms about the situation. For scientists, this uncertainty—as seen in Castuera case—was implicit in the nature of the archaeological work performed in the context of war and postwar mass burial sites. For the archaeologist, the repressive pattern that the archive evoked (i.e., the killing of such a large group at once) was rare, as her experience in previous exhumations of similar nature had shown that the so-called *sacas* were realized in smaller numbers and on different days. As the team continued working further down the trench line, another group of eight bodies appeared. The disparity and contradictions between neighbours' assumptions, archival data, and the reality that the mass grave expounded provoked people's insecurity, for some established inferences about the killings had been overturned. As José reflected during an interview after the exhumation had taken place:

> I even thought we would not find what we were looking for. When we found another [group of] eight and so there were sixteen, I thought [the excavation] was going to finish there. I thought it would finish there because we were not sure about where the trench ended, for according to elders, it ceased before what we then saw. I thought: if I have the death certificates of 26 or 27 [men], we are missing 12. When I saw this I was *stunned.* (José Sánchez-Paniagua, Puebla, 2012)

The unexpected content of the mass grave made José feel at a loss. In this situation, archaeologists decided to open the whole of the trench, mainly, in Laura's words, for the "families' peace of mind." As archaeological labour progressed, however, more groups were located along the first trench (TR1). Four groups, each containing the human remains of 8 to 10 individuals, were found in the area of *El Chaparral.* Likewise, a group of 12 was later encountered in another trench (named TR2 in the archaeological record) in *Cuesta de la Cabeza.* Through the stories of neighbours, archaeologists had been able to understand some of the events recorded in the mass grave, invoked by the corpses and their disposition. For neighbours, on the other hand, archaeological practice provided a source of confirmation or negation of the stories they knew. For instance, when the first trench (TR1) and the second trench (TR2) were unearthed, numerous corpses emerged severed and bore no anatomic connection between their body parts. This situation occurred in every archaeologically-delineated zone in the two trenches. In each area, piles of scattered bones and objects, where legs, arms and skulls were amalgamated in a chaotic disposition, appeared next to discarded limbs, bodily fragments, and incomplete skeletons. These dispersed parts, which were labelled "de-contextualized" in scientific argot or described in neighbours' observations as "ramshackle," (Fig 5.2) summoned the image of wild rabbits, dogs, or wolves "pulling them out," as recalled by some accounts. For archaeologists, the exposure of the bodies spoke of the exemplary meaning of these killings in the specific postwar milieu (see also Renshaw 2011). For families, the tangle of human remains made this lurid part of the story evident and shocking. These muddled remnants, which could only be recomposed into a coherent whole by the physical anthropologist, became, once again, as in Castuera case, a testimony (Domanska 2005, 403) of the damage caused by vermin to the bodies' physiognomy.

In Castuera, scientific evidence confirmed the functioning of the Camp in a world of uncertain historical data and instilled hope in connection to the inconclusive searches for disappeared kin. In Puebla, the scientific finding of the mass graves challenged a deep-rooted social and familial knowledge about the executions that had been part of the experience of different generations. In his study of how the Merina in Madagascar experience history, Maurice Bloch (1996) has argued that the group shares a dual perception of a person, which leads them to conceive history as both a changing and static practice. Drawing on philosophical ideas from Plato and Aristotle on the understanding of the external or internal constructions of memory, Bloch argues that whether the Merina conceive events in history as something that transforms a person during her young life—"endlessly modified by the moment and the imprint these moments leave on it" (ibid., 227)—at old age and through burial, the person becomes immortalized, securing their permanence in their social group. History is thus understood as a fluid process in which the individual is immersed throughout life and comes to a fixed state near death, which secures social regeneration, kinship ties, and traceable genealogies.

In a similar sense, one could argue that in Puebla, the overarching presence of some mnemonic accounts, their frequent retelling and recurrence among some families and members in relation to the suffering of their ancestors, provided some stories with strong fact-like qualities and an immobile character, thus asserting people's "shared historicity" (Skultans 1998; Fabian 1983) and their own kinship genealogy. Confronted by the opened mass graves, well-established familiar narratives about the killings, passed on by members of previous generations or through hearsay, became perturbed and unsettled. The sight of these corpses and their scientific interpretation became important elements

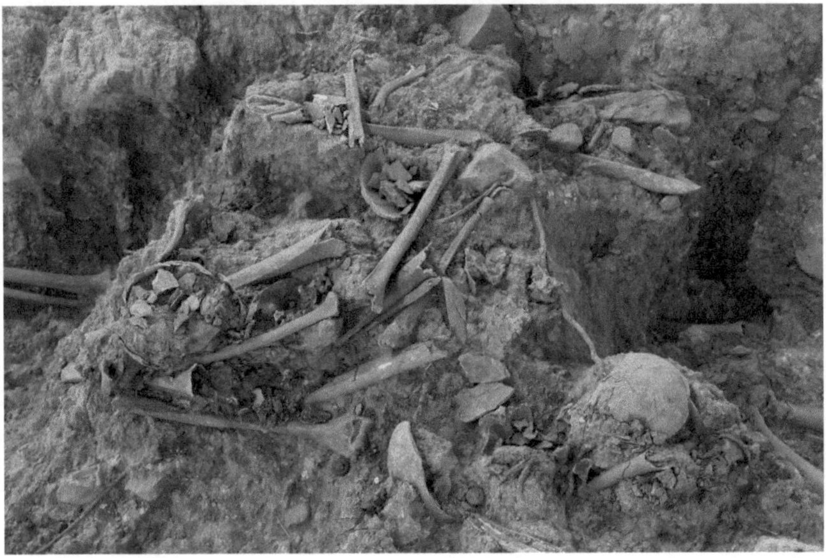

Fig. 5.2 Second group of bones with no anatomical connection found in Trench no 1 (TR1)

in the negotiation of new meanings about the executions, which were adopted by relatives and neighbours throughout the exhumation. Such a process of substantiation pressed people to confront a different perception of their own history, as it validated some stories and turned others into myths.

One day at the graveside, José's sister Consuelo Sánchez-Paniagua, her husband, Antonio, and Mariano and José, the grandsons of Mariano Gómez Mayoral, one of the men buried in the mass grave, discussed the authenticity of a widespread rumour that spawned in the village in the wake of the murders. During the exhumation, many neighbours retold in different forms the story that some of the men taken to the trenches might have survived the execution and escaped. Some believed this to be true—on occasions retelling full stories about the vicissitudes these men underwent during the years they spent in hiding. Others categorically denied the incident. In a long conversation about the executions, when Mariano hinted at the event of the likely escape of one of these men, the rest of the group argued for the impossibility of this having happened, referring to the materials found in the mass grave as evidence contesting the rumour. Arguing that they had all been given a "kill shot" (*tiro de gracia*) after the execution and that they had been firmly tied by the wrists and arms to one another—in a similar manner to the bodies found in Castuera. Consuelo and Antonio, who followed the development of the team's work daily, decidedly referenced the objects of the mass graves to sustain their claim:

Mariano: Maybe some could have escaped…

Antonio: No, they didn't, they received kill shots. They came back to finish them off.

Consuelo: Don't you see that a Muga was wounded…

Antonio: They are all tied! From here and from here [pointing at wrists and forearms] according to Laura…

Consuelo: Besides, they are there! [Pointing at the mass grave]

In contrast to the cases described in the previous chapter, where objects contributed to the imagination of the death of a relative and their identity, here it was the traces of violence found on the skeletons that superseded survival and ghostly visions of families in the past. For two other relatives, Jacinto and Begoña Velasco Sánchez-Paniagua, the killing of their grandfather, Pelayo Velasco, was surrounded by rumours about his possible escape from the site, as some people told the family he had only been wounded in an eye and had later been healed by someone in the countryside. Begoña ascertained that it was her grandfather's sister "who later started the rumour," for she stated she had once seen him working in a cafe in San Sebastian, in northern Spain. Begoña and Jacinto's grandmother, the siblings explained, never believed this because she was sure that her husband would have returned home, had he been alive.

For Pablo Trenado Cabanillas, another relative who lost his grandfather, Mariano Cabanillas López, and uncle, Felipe Cabanillas Herrera—two leather workers who made packsaddles for draft animals—his mother's hope, conversely, was that his brother Felipe "would have survived." When some neighbours went to bury the men killed, they assured Pablo's mother that the bodies of Felipe and another man were not in the mass grave. Later on, when the family moved to Madrid,

Pablo recalled, his mother thought she saw him in a flea market and later on the streets, although Pablo himself never believed his uncle was alive. These predicaments over a likely escape reflected the different ways in which grieving relatives dealt with such uncertainty, as in Castuera. When Begoña visited the mass grave, however, she was impressed. For her, seeing the corpses and the cable wire, "confirm[ed] that [her] grandfather could not have escaped" (Begoña Velasco, Puebla, 2012). Pablo also doubted it when he saw "the way they were tied" (Pablo Trenado Cabanillas, Puebla, 2012). As in the case of the mass graves excavated in Castuera, the cables used to join the prisoners, tightly knotted with a navy technique (as recognized by one of the archaeologists) enraptured visitors and provoked an emotional reaction. Their sombre presence pushed inner reworkings of a family's past.

Discussions by the graveside also reflected an ongoing concern with figures. Many of the neighbours who gathered around the mass graves often deliberated about the number of people killed and their identities, tracing a genealogy of the men whilst devising their common kinship relations. For years, many had argued that more men were killed in *Cuesta de la Cabeza* than in the lower area of *El Chaparral.* Some spoke of forty, others eighty, and even hundreds of deaths. Forty-two bodies were eventually exhumed in Puebla, of which thirty were found in *El Chaparral* and twelve in *Cuesta de la Cabeza.* Nonetheless, the total number of people who died as a result of Francoist repression in Puebla—counting those executed in other towns and prisons—amounted to more than 120 people. The controversies derived from a need to prove the ferocity of Francoist repression in this localized scenario and, as in Castuera, in contraposition to the number of right-wing dead in Puebla—thirty-seven men from right-wing families, as neighbours explained, were killed at the start of the war in the village. Talking about numbers also led people to articulate the names of some of those in the mass grave.

Some of the stories heard from those who had witnessed the creation of the mass grave or lived the event firsthand, as in the case of a man called Mariano, nicknamed "Conejo" (Rabbit), exemplified the way in which the identity of some of the dead men had travelled as part of the most enduring memories. In an interview carried out with Mariano next to the mass grave, he reminisced about a time when he, aged 13, and two other friends went to inspect the mass grave days after the killings had taken place. He remembered the hats—"we saw many hats stained with blood", he ascertained—and recognized one man, Vicente Muga—who was killed together with his brother and father—by the "jacket he was wearing". Many other stories made reference to the way in which other people also identified their relatives in the grave. José's grandmother, for instance, had identified her husband, according to Consuelo, also "by his jacket's lining" when she ventured to hastily cover up the bodies. These forms of identification, socially recalled in many oral accounts, evoked a dislocated recognition of the body through a materiality nearly lost inside the mass grave in the present. Mainly durable fragments of garments, such as buttons, shoe soles, zips or a safety pin, among other personal objects, remained existent at the time of the exhumation.

The scarce number of objects in both trenches made the archaeologists' work of identification more complicated, as their absence limited the possibility of delineating a personal profile for the victim. In Puebla, in contrast to Mass Grave 1 in Castuera, only a few significant belongings that could be salient for a presumptive identification were found. Objects such as a medal, a set of pieces carved out of tiles to play a game (depicted on the cover image of this book), or a pair of scissors threw some light on to whom the human remains of each individual might have belonged—however, not enough to enable a full identification. To the issue that not all the families of those believed to be in the mass grave could be contacted (some were no longer traceable) or that other relatives chose not to get involved in the exhumation (something often criticized by the families who visited the site), one had to add, again, the bad conservation of the bones in some zones of TR1 and TR2. In some areas, many of the bones had effectively turned into dust. The prospect of the positive identification of most of these skeletons thus became faint and scientists relied heavily on accounts from direct witnesses that provided physical and personal details, which aided recognition of the individuals inside the grave. Family and neighbours' accounts retraced the memory of the defeated, unfolding clues about their physiognomy, occupation, and habits, as well as about their personalities, village and kin relations, and their political affiliations. Testimonies could estimate an identity and also point to the cause of the death, enabling Laura's historical analysis of repression in this part of the region.

Identifying the Familial Body

I was entrusted with gathering interviews to help the team to collect archaeological and anthropological information about the corpses and their deaths and to map the social relationships woven around the mass grave. The formulation of interview questions, however, was an ongoing collaborative effort between archaeologists and social anthropologists. When I spoke to witnesses or relatives of the men executed, questions about the individual's age, pathologies, customs, or professional occupation mixed with descriptions about these men's political activities, their social role within the village's networks, or the family's intimate experience of their arrest and execution. Interviews and conversations with those eager to share their version of the events made the act of recollection significant, not only for the value of what was said—which spoke of the personal traits of the deceased—but also for the relation established with the past through telling—which unravelled aspects about the identity of the storyteller in the present.

Questions that aimed to collect information that could be contrasted with the materiality of the mass grave demanded an ingrained understanding of the physical condition of the executed, as well as his lifestyle or aspects of the moment of his death on the part of the relative. When José and Consuelo, for instance, described the story of their grandfather, they recounted how, just before he was executed, he was taken for interrogation and during the questioning someone broke most of his teeth with the butt of a rifle. This retelling, which was painfully undertaken by the siblings, showed the emotional affliction the event had caused in the family. Retelling it, however, was intimately connected to the mass grave, as trails of the story could have been found in the bones, had they been in better condition. Moreover, my interview also included questions about these men's possessions or what they had at the time of their death, for such objects could appear in the mass grave. As it turned out, however, most men carried little with them. In José's grandfather's case, whilst being in jail, he gave his pocket watch to his sister, Escolastia, during one of her visits to the village prison. As both brother and sister recalled, knowing he would soon die, he left his last possession to his family—just as Aurora Navas's mother did before she was killed in Castuera. His wish was for his son José—Consuelo and José's father—to look after it. José, at a later age, would give it to his son with the same purpose. When José (the son) spoke to me about the family's past at his house on various occasions, the watch was taken out and shown, as another fragment through which the story was articulated.

Sarah Wagner (2008) has observed how, often, during ante-mortem interviews, memory can play tricks on respondents, making them mistake traits of the missing person or forget personal details altogether (2008, 133). In Puebla, decades after the conflict and bearing only the information they had learnt, other second- and third-generation relatives did not know much about the objects or clothing their kin might have worn when they died. Some speculated that they probably did not have many belongings, as some had been taken straight from their houses in the middle of the night or after a day's work, or could have been searched if they had been imprisoned—back in the mass grave, the appearance of spoons suggested, like in the Camp, that some men could have spent, in fact, days in jail. Many relatives hence kept scarce information about their kin's belongings or physical attributes. For instance, the brothers Mariano and José, grandsons of Mariano Gómez Mayoral, kept only an image of their grandfather. Likewise, Begoña and Jacinto Velasco's family had preserved only a wooden barrel built by their grandfather, Pelayo, and a picture of him at a young age. The existence of images of the men executed in some families' archives prompted José to collect them for his own historical inquiry. Likewise, these old images, sometimes taken with a camera and sometimes painted on canvas, became also an important element in the process of archaeological and anthropological assembly. In the absence of firsthand descriptions of their physiognomy, these images enabled the depiction of a face and a body that aided the imagination of the person by scientists and neighbours alike, even if bones and skulls were badly damaged by erosion in the mass graves.

Family records also provided other images in which some appeared in a different disposition and situation. As opposed to the portraits, which showed most men in classical individual profile and full view, posed or otherwise, in groups in a studio or in the village's streets (see Fig. 5.3), other images, such as Fig. 5.4, evoked a political sentiment, bringing the ideological past of some of those in the mass grave closer to present generations. Figure 5.4 shows a group of neighbours from Puebla standing and sitting outside the old branch of the *Unión General de Trabajadores* or UGT (General Worker's Union), the trade union with affiliated militants in the village. The image is part of Sofía Sierra's collection, the daughter of Baltasar Expósito Sierra (as known in the municipal and civil registry[4]), a shoemaker from Puebla de Alcocer also killed and buried in 1939 in *Bodegones*. The same image was also part of Esperanza Muga's family archive. Esperanza was the daughter of Rafael Muga Ruiz, a tradesman also killed in the *sacas* of the spring of 1939.

Sofía and Esperanza's families had given the image to José to aid his historical investigation into the executions. The photograph, as Sofía's

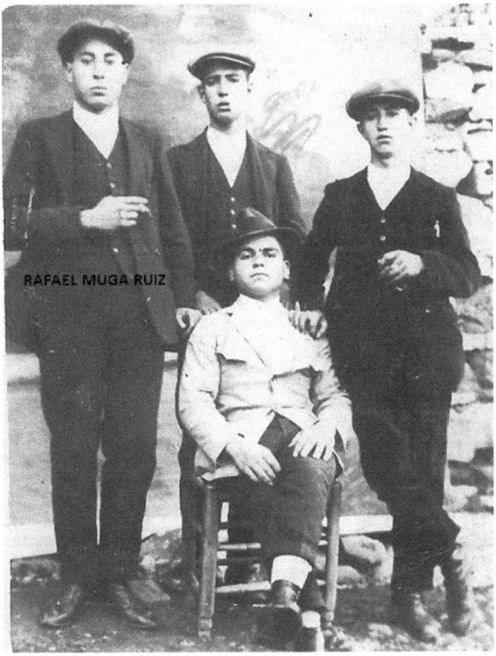

Fig. 5.3 Picture of Rafael Muga Ruiz with other men. Courtesy of Esperanza Muga and José Sánchez-Paniagua

son-in-law explained to me when he visited the exhumation with Sofía's daughter in August 2012, was taken in 1929 and shows Baltasar sitting on the left hand corner of the table, accompanied by other men and women connected to the union, with his left fist raised. Rafael Muga Ruiz, Esperanza's father, is sitting on the right hand corner, reading a newspaper. He also appears in Fig. 5.3, identified by his name, which is typed where he stands. As his daughter Esperanza recounted in an interview, Rafael was killed with his father, also called Rafael, and his brother Vicente. Esperanza believes the three of them were killed because of the position another brother, Eugenio, held as the socialist (PSOE) town mayor of Puebla during the war, from 1936 until 1939. Eugenio was also killed by court-martial in April 1940 in the city of Mérida.

Moreover, although I never had the chance to interview Baltasar's daughter, Sofía, as her delicate health did not allow her to come from Madrid, where she lived, to the exhumation, many people commented on Baltasar's death to me at the gravesite. Some described how he disappeared after a fellow neighbour invited him to have a coffee from

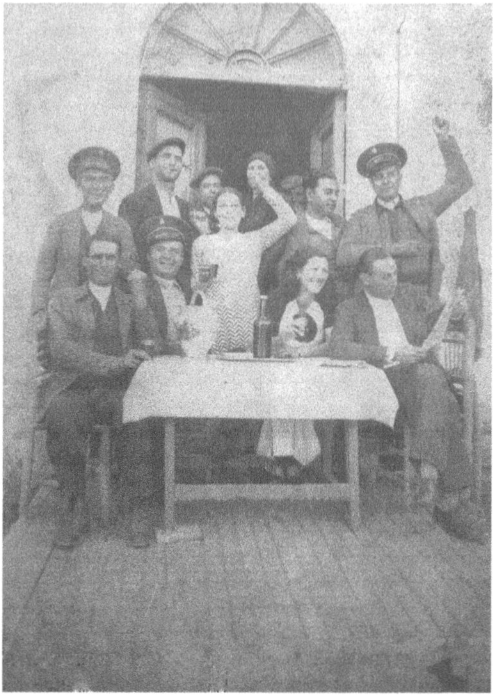

Fig. 5.4 Picture of neighbours from Puebla outside the UGT branch Courtesy of Esperanza Muga, and José Sánchez-Paniagua

which he never returned. Emilio, Sofia's son-in-law, explained to me that Baltasar held an influential position within the trade union (UGT). According to him, all the people in the photograph were killed or repressed in some way after the war ended, suggesting that Baltasar's death, like many others, was politically motivated. The image provided a peek into an otherwise only imagined political past—that is at times also eluded by some families, sharpening the outline of these social identities and bringing them back into focus (Hirsch 2008, 2012).

Indeed, traces of these men's political identities, embodied in captured gestures, as in the case of Fig. 5.4, or in the oral accounts that remained, were often invoked in people's mnemonic exchanges. Broken accounts offered a brief encounter, like a Proustian involuntary flash, into their political and social aspirations, composing a fuzzy history of the relations between left- and right-wing groups of neighbours before, during, and after the war. These narratives turned the dead men into characters through which the theatre of confrontations and social unrest existing at the time, in the village, unfolded. The biographical stories people told at the gravesite—but also in the closeness of their living rooms, during some of our interviews—often hinted at a broader context in which national and local histories were entwined (Pine 2007; Skultans 1998). Through the stories that were shared between families and researchers and among family members, firsthand and learnt memories situated the mass grave and the bodies in a pre-war and war milieu, sketching not only individual traits but also a historical topography, in which the particularities of the repression in the area were delineated. This was essential for Laura's "diachronic reading of the mass grave" (informal conversation with Laura Muñoz Encinar 2014) in which local events were considered in relation to other cases in the region.

Many relatives' tellings of their kin's past, just like in Fig. 5.4, associated these life accounts with their political involvement in a period of intense class conflict. In a joint interview with José and Consuelo Sánchez-Paniagua and their father José—who is affected by Parkinson's disease—the first two helped their relative to recall aspects of his father's active participation in village politics during the Second Republic. Consuelo recounted how her grandfather, Pedro Sánchez-Paniagua, was a miner who founded the *Casa del Pueblo* or People's House, where workers from different left-wing groups gathered for meetings. José's father described this as "the place where the poor met to talk about their things." Historian Fernando Sánchez Marroyo (1990) has located the emergence and rise of these institutions in the 1920s. These places, according to Marroyo, "were used as headquarters for diverse trading societies and they were the centre for the irradiation of the associative influence in general and socialist influence in particular" (1990, 128) in such rural enclaves. According to his relatives, Pedro Sánchez-Paniagua also created a student music group, who sometimes serenaded the rich, singing critical songs that challenged their favourable position in village society. Some of these songs, as José's father recalled, chanted for the "bread, work, and freedom of workers." José, his son, and his daughter identified his active political commitment to the interests of Puebla's working class as one of the main causes of his murder.

It is important to note that the lives and deaths of these men were intimately entangled with a social conflict that also affected the region and country more generally. These tensions, as Francisco Espinosa Maestre (2007) has pointed out, were profoundly determined, among other things, by the crisis around land distribution and the consequences brought about by the Land Reform Law of 1931, which produced an open-ended brawl between farmers and landowners up until the outbreak of the war in 1936. Many of the measures promoted by the new law—regarding labour costs, hiring and working conditions, and land expropriation—enraged landowners, who saw their capital privileges being threatened and their personalities undermined, especially in Extremadura. Land workers' collectives, who mostly adhered to socialist ideas in the province of Badajoz, for their part, soon grew disillusioned with the slow transformation of workers' rights over the land (locked in the hands of a few), promised by the first left-wing coalition government of the Second Republic (Espinosa 2007). This led to a growing sense of discontent—as poverty and unemployment grew among the working classes. Social despair led to the emergency occupation and settlement of privately owned terrains by some farming groups, especially ploughmen (Riesco 2006), during the first *Bienio Reformista* (Reformist Period).

From 1933 and with the start of the conservative *Bienio Negro* (Black Two Years) that would last until 1936, the repression of the worker's movement by landowners and right-wing parties alike was widely felt on a micro level. In Puebla, for instance, the Socialist Association was dissolved in 1933, as part of the restraining campaigns of the government all over the province, which closed down many *Casas del Pueblo* and suppressed workers' initiatives more generally (Espinosa 2007, 65). In a village where over 54% of the inhabitants were farmers (mostly ploughmen, day labourers, guest farm workers or sharecroppers), according to José, one can imagine the difficult situation lived between different social groups. Some like Espinosa (ibid.) have shown that the efforts made in the run up to the general election of 1936 by all political organizations indicated that much was at stake after these tumultuous periods of reform and counter reform. The election of 1936 became decisive for left- and right-wing collectives and votes, as the historian suggests. In the particular case of Puebla de Alcocer, Espinosa cites the example of the village's Land Registrar, originally from Mérida, who though not inscribed in the list of registered voters, nevertheless imposed his ballot for the right-wing party *Acción Popular* (ibid., 94) at the voting desk. In our interview, Pablo Trenado Cabanillas explained how he believed his grandfather, Mariano Cabanillas López, and uncle, Felipe Cabanillas Herrera, were killed because his grandfather refused to sell his family's votes to right-wing neighbours—presumably prior to the general election of 1936. In his story, Pablo explains how his grandfather, of socialist ideas, had "nine children and so their votes were worth a lot" (Pablo Trenado Cabanillas, Puebla, 2012). According to Pablo, they killed his grandfather and uncle because of these political clashes.

Pablo acknowledges that the subject of the war and killings were, in his words, "taboo" in his household. Though his mother had recounted to him how men from the village took father and son from their beds while they were sleeping, the reason for their execution remained unclear to him. Pablo's family's history of extreme repression needs to be understood within the framework of the abovementioned political intricacies. Apart from Pablo's father Mariano and brother Felipe, two more of Mariano's sons, Luis and Pedro, were killed in other cities of the province by court-martial and three of his daughters jailed—first in Puebla, and later in a prison in the Basque Country. Pablo's mother, Agustina, was one of them. According to him, his mother was also imprisoned "for giving her vote to the socialists." Doubtlessly, as Pablo retold his story, one could perceive the connections between the fragments he recalled from transmitted accounts and the bleary village reality archaeologists and I, members of a later generation, began to discern in relation to other experiences and historical records gathered as the exhumation advanced. Pablo and José's accounts hence needed to be threaded with the information that other neighbours from older generations provided about past disputes and in the context of a pre-war society.

When talking to other neighbours, especially those from older generations, many ascertained that the roots of the conflict between right- and left-wing neighbours could be traced back to clashes that occurred between landowners and workers over a terrain that was commonly owned by the village but later sold to private owners, after the war, known as the *Casa Carrasco*. Some of the older witnesses who remembered what happened suggested that problems with this plot caused many of the deaths in the village when the war started. In an interview with Emiliano Bayón Villarejo, a 95-year-old man who was an adolescent during the years of the Second Republic in Puebla and worked the fields with his father as a ploughman, he remembered well the moment when, aged 14, and after the Land Reform was approved, "things got better for workers." Labour, he reminisced, was more abundant and paid more generously, especially as many farmers benefited from the partition of some landowner's untouched large estates, rented out as part of the government's plan for agricultural intensification (Espinosa 2007).[5] In Puebla, Emiliano remembered, the expropriation of *Casa Carrasco* was a trigger for later confrontations between neighbours. According to Emiliano's account and others, neighbours from the village "knocked down the walls" of the plot to claim it back during the Second Republic. It is not clear to me from people's stories whether the plot was occupied as a result of the process of collectivisation propelled by the new Land Reform in 1931, which aimed to re-distribute common property privatized as a result of the Spanish *desamortización* or liberal agrarian reform from the 18th to the early years of the 20th century (ibid.)[6], or whether this occurred at a later stage, at the outset of the conflict. As Emiliano remembered:

> They said that the *Casa Carrasco* had always belonged to all people in the village. When the Movement broke out—I remember it was during the Republic—people went there and they knocked down the walls. There were many people and they knocked the walls down. That cost plenty of deaths… that and the plot… The *Casa Carrasco* was the cause of the majority of the deaths there [at the mass grave]. Because there were people who thought that that [land] was not theirs [the landowners'], that it had been bought with fake witnesses and so on… And it brought many, many deaths and politics too. When the Movement broke out, it was people's land and during the Republic, since the first election I knew, when Azaña's government won—the first Republican president—the *Casa Carrasco* was knocked to the ground and all the people in the village had their animals there… (Emiliano Bayón Villarejo, Entrerríos, 2012)

Stories depicted the allotment as a grazing land where neighbours could keep their livestock for a small fee paid to the town hall. As Mariano "Conejo" explained to me "whoever had a cow or mare […] or sheep would put them there because it was the village's plot." According to him, most villagers participated in the "knock down of *Casa Carrasco*," as he referred to it. It seems that during the Second Republic neighbours enjoyed *Casa Carrasco* as a common property until, as Emiliano implied above, the "Movement" (Francoist uprising) broke out. It was in those years, Mariano also claimed, when "right-wing lawyers and public notaries appropriated the land", dividing it among a few well-to-do neighbours from Puebla. It is also not clear from my interviews and notes what the direct relation was between this widely-observed event and the executions of the men in the mass grave (e.g., who participated and were involved in the occupation and eviction of the land). Most of these narratives were broken, for temporal distance contravened some of these witnesses' mnemonic recollection—this was also often acknowledged by second generation kin, who recognized the discontinuities in some elder's narratives. It was apparent that the repressive acts recalled in Puebla were set against this background of land and political disputes; however, there was no trace of these events in the municipal archive, as José explained to me—since most of the archival files prior to 1939 had been burnt or destroyed in an effort on the part of Republican authorities to protect neighbours when the war was lost. José, whose research into the executions led him to reconstruct parts of the pre-war archive, had not been able to find town hall minutes or any notes about the "*knock down*" in any of the regional depositories he consulted. He could only obtain documents about the moment the property was bought in 1942, when the terrain was privatized and later partitioned for renting. The discord over the *Casa Carrasco* would remain enigmatic and only present in the memory of elders and younger generations who had learnt faint details about the expropriation.

Working with some of these firsthand oral histories often entailed piecing together distinct incidents in order to understand the nature of the killings. For instance, Emiliano also thought these deaths were an act of retaliation for the detention and assassination of 37 right-wing neighbours in Puebla in 1937. One could infer from his words that the issue of ownership over the plot also triggered the killings perpetrated by the left at the beginning of the war: "they should have not killed them, there was no reason for it, it all happened because of the *Casa Carrasco* . . . because others said they [landowners] took things that were not theirs" (Emiliano Bayón Villarejo, Entrerríos, 2012). Elders' stories described how some left-wing villagers had gathered inside the church to elaborate a list of right-wing counterparts and vote on whether they should be killed. According to Emiliano, when the power shifted to Francoist authorities after the war, right-wing neighbours and those who then supported the new regime arrested and killed most of the men who were in the mass graves in an act of revenge. This cause-and-effect relation remains fuzzy. Nonetheless, the connection that people make between both murders elucidate how, for some, speaking about the killings of those in the grave meant evoking these other dead—whose pervasiveness was manifested in the way they had been rehashed through these narratives and materialised through the carved names imprinted and commemorated at the bottom the Cross of the Fallen, next to the church's courtyard, since the postwar period (Fig. 5.5).

Fig. 5.5 Cross of the fallen, Puebla de Alcocer

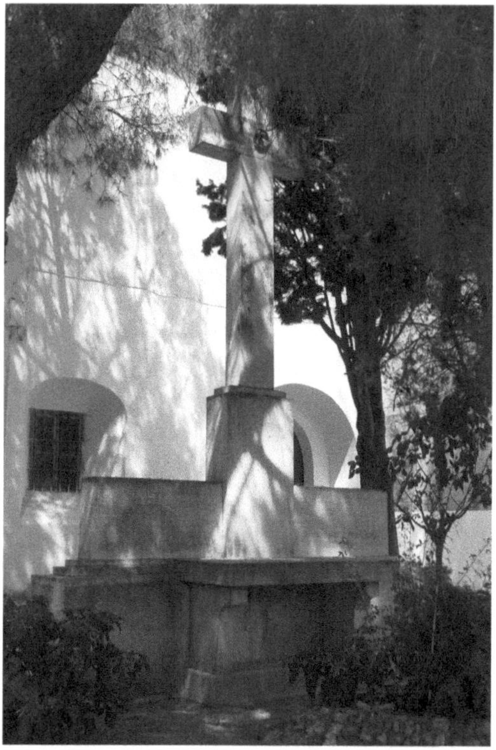

Some stories had survived in people's imagination for the fascination they awakened within the community, turning some of their protagonists into referents of narratives of Republican loss in Puebla. A case in point is the figure of Esperanza Muga's uncle, Eugenio Muga Ruiz, whose role as town mayor during the years of the war was widely invoked in accounts given by neighbours but also family relatives. Executed by firing squad after a court martial celebrated in Mérida in 1940, some elders spoke of Muga as a revolutionary man, who helped to spread socialist ideas in nearby villages and around the province; people like Muga, as Sánchez Marroyo (1990) has observed, were key in the expansion of the socialist movement in the region. Some elders' narratives identified the town mayor as the instigator of the killings of the right-wing detainees in 1937, ascertaining that the remorseless treatment he and his relatives received after the war ended was a consequence of his mandate as socialist town leader. His life and death story were haunting for the extreme violence he and his family members endured. When Muga was arrested in the village in the aftermath of the conflict, he was jailed and beaten before being taken to Mérida to be prosecuted. Three other members of the Muga family, namely his father Rafael and two other brothers, Rafael and Vicente, were killed during the same period and buried in the trenches of *Bodegones*. Muga's biography was entangled with his family's painful fate, often retold by visitors who confronted the grave and the potential remains of the three men it contained.

At the mass grave, people depicted the moment when, after the execution, one of the brothers, Vicente—the person Mariano "Conejo" would recognize inside the mass grave days after the execution, still alive, called for his father ("Father, father!"), attracting the attention of the perpetrators, who returned and "finished them off," as Consuelo and her husband Antonio recounted. The Muga's history of violence also evoked other death stories. One of the most frequently recited accounts was that connected to Muga's partner, Maria Quiteria, with whom Muga had a child. Nearly every visitor that came to the site repeated, in the same sequential order, the details of her ghastly death. The story of Maria Quiteria was known across generations, exposing the affective potency of these postwar violent episodes in the articulation of a social history of suffering in the village. As most versions agreed, Maria Quiteria was also taken to prison at the end of the war, where she waited to obtain the endorsement of a right-wing family friend, which would grant her release. According to neighbours, the night before her reprieve arrived, her killer, knowing her acquittal was under way, took her out of prison to execute her. As villagers explained, three right-wing neighbours from the village led her to the cemetery accompanied by members of the military.

In the testimony of Esperanza Muga, the daughter of Eugenio Muga's brother, Rafael, she attributed her family's adversity first of all to the envy others felt of her family's prosperity before the war—highlighting her grandfathers' blooming tobacco shop or her uncles' access to education. Nonetheless, later in our conversation, Esperanza recognized that her father's death was directly connected to the role her uncle had as the socialist town mayor of Puebla de Alcocer during the war. She mentioned on several occasions that the family did not go into exile in France since they didn't think anything would happen to them, for it was only Eugenio who held a political position. Ascribing the motive for her family's killing to material envy or the political ideology of her uncle resembled a move to depoliticise—whether consciously or unconsciously—her kin's past, as authors like Leyla Renshaw (2011) have argued occurred in other Spanish contexts. Indeed, this obscurity around Esperanza's father's political identity could be interpreted as a consequence of a postwar reality where Republican political ideals became hazardous and harshly punished. It could also be understood as the result of the family's silence around some aspects of her father's death. Esperanza's frail memories stood in contrast to the image of Fig. 5.4, where her father reads the paper on the doorstep of the branch of UGT in the village, surrounded by other trade unionists.

The stories collected in Puebla during the exhumation spoke of the way in which living memories from first generations and learnt accounts from younger generations were turned into a form of data, in order to gain historical "depth" with regard to the executions. Andrew Lass (1994) has pointed out in his study about the making of history in Czechoslovakia after the events of 17th November 1989 (or the "Velvet Revolution") how individual memory became an important element in the creation of collective representations of the event. In so doing, Lass argues, individual actors became active historical agents, who through lived personal narratives and the appropriation of others' recollections (e.g., in memoirs and other cultural products) crafted formalized histories. In Puebla, relatives and villagers' life histories came to be active traces in the composition of the temporal sequence of the killings. In the process, however, and as Lass also observes in an indirect manner, these narratives also reasserted specific political positions and opened a common ideological bond that some children and grandchildren felt with their kin and other personalities of the village. Some, like Esperanza, expressed this subtly, for example when she hinted at her unconditional voting for the socialist party over the years. Others purposely established a genealogical link with their relatives' socialist ideology, as something that "runs in the family" or that they were born with. For many, ideology was congenital, accentuating the commonalities between kin not only through the physical attributes that scientific praxis sought in the formulation of a positive identification but also through a sense of a shared morality and worldview.

On some occasions, this continuity between past and present identities was accentuated when discussing the consequences of the conflict, for instance when some pointed out "*We* also killed people!"—assimilating a timeless political connection. In this regard, these men's political identities were also connected to the profound antagonisms that, still in 2012, existed between right- and left-wing neighbours and which many neighbours talked about at the exhumation. The at-times cautious or more explicit commitment to a socialist ideology on the part of relatives made these corpses very much part of the village's socio-political present. Ideological connections between present and past generations were often claimed on the basis of blood kinship, as something inherited and passed on. This provided the mass grave and its exhumation with a sacred character—just as it had acquired for the *political family* of activists in Castuera. In both scenarios, the exhumation and the stories shared connected the living and the dead across a temporal divide (Cruikshank 1998; Fabian 1983).

In the context of Puebla, familial and neighbourly stories elucidated the way in which these deaths had secretly lived on as part of private acts of transmission between generations. The collective imagination formed about the killings, through interaction between local stories and archaeological evidence, was fraught with particular uncertainties over the murders and their mediation—as archaeological reasoning entered the social history of the village. The act of retelling the past aided archaeologists in understanding the story of these deaths, but also helped them to contextualize, in relation to other histories and archival records, the intricacies of the executions in *Bodegones*. The unearthing of the human remains, however, was also marked by the way in which the corpses had haunted generations after the war and until the exhumation. The production of historical knowledge through the practice of exhumation is deeply imbued with the subjective experience of these killings and the trauma of different generations. To study these forms of history-making is to examine their emotional, sensual, and emotive worlds, which are forged by facts about the haunting violence of the killings and the pain and suffering they provoked. The story of death and disappearance in Puebla or Castuera is not solely contained in the past of the executions but expands into the lives and histories of the living, eliciting the affective strength of these deaths in the shaping of collective and individual experiences of violence.

Notes

1. During the postwar years, with the implementation of the so-called *Plan Badajoz*, many families were given a plot of land and some livestock in different locations, prompting the formation of new villages—called commonly "colonization towns"—all around the province. According to the town mayor, around 200 families emigrated from Puebla to a new area where these plots were located. There, they built the new village, *Entrerríos*, from scratch. Many of the families that left were families associated with the left-wing Republican past of the village.
2. For some archaeological experts working in the field of exhumations—among them Laura Muñoz Encinar—this technique seems to lack reliability, as it often offers contradictory and vague information about the burials, failing, on many occasions, to determine whether in fact there are or are not human remains in the areas examined. Experts such as Muñoz Encinar do not consider this technological device to have a particularly high success rate in relation to mass burial location—at least in connection to cases in Extremadura (personal communication with Laura Muñoz Encinar).
3. On an occasion, this became problematic for José, as a neighbour, presumably of right-wing affiliation, had told a well-to-do family of Puebla, after he had visited the site, that another neighbour interviewed at the gravesite had slandered the family. José, saddened and angry, spoke to the concerned family to clarify that what they had heard was an unfounded claim. He would later also confront the man who created the rumour, calling him a "liar," whilst the man responded that he was unsure about where he had heard the rumour or who had told him about it at the excavation site.
4. When the family visited the exhumation, they said his surname "Éxposito" was a surprise to them, for he had always used "Sierra". "Sierra" is also the name that was passed on to his offspring and to later generations. "Éxposito" was a name that they did not recognize as theirs, and this triggered a sense of bewilderment over their relative's identity, registry, and life history.
5. Sergio Riesco (2006) has noted that many other ploughmen who did not benefit from what was commonly known as "la agraria" (Land Reform Law) constituted an active group of land petitioners and a strong occupying force, which led to the non-violent invasion of private plots from 1932. Their demands would be felt then and again after the election of 1936, when another intense wave of invasions occurred (ibid.).
6. The process of *desamortización* aimed to privatize many of the properties held for centuries by the Church, signitories, nobility, and municipal institutions, with a clear economic and political purpose, as Espinosa points out

(2007, 17). There were two important stages in the process of *desamortización*, one led by Medizábal in 1836, mainly of Church properties and by Madoz in 1855, of a civil character. In Extremadura, as Espinosa observes, citing Juan García Pérez, the *desamortización* "meant the transfer of around one and a half a million hectares to private owners" (Espinosa Maestre 2007, 18). Large estates were acquired by a reduced number of owners, who "opted for a profitable and safe agrarian capitalism around pasture as the unit of production" (ibid.). Such an oligarchic regime persisted until the start of the Second Republic in 1931.

References

Bloch, Maurice. 1996. Internal and External Memory: Different Ways of Being in History. In *Tense Past: Cultural Essays in Trauma and Memory*, ed. Michael Lambeck, and Paul Antze. London: Routledge.

Boyarin, Jonathan. 1994. *Remapping Memory: The Politics of Timespace*. Minneapolis: University of Minnesota Press.

Burke, Peter. 1989. History as Social Memory. In *Memory, History, Culture, and the Mind*, ed. Thomas Butler. Oxford: Basil Blackwell.

Cruikshank, Julie. 1998. *The Social Life of Stories: Narrative and Knowledge in the Yukon Territory*. Lincoln: University of Nebraska Press.

Cruikshank, Julie. 2005. *Do Glaciers Listen? Local Knowledge, Colonial Encounters, and Social Imagination*. Canada: University of British Columbia Press.

Domanska, Ewa. 2005. Toward the Archaeontology of the Dead Body. *Rethinking History* 9 (4): 389–413.

Espinosa Maestre, Francisco. 2007. *La primavera del Frente Popular: los campesinos de Badajoz y el origen de la Guerra Civil (marzo-julio de 1936)*. Barcelona: Crítica.

Fabian, Johannes. 1983. *Time and the Other: How Anthropology Makes its Object*. New York: Columbia University Press.

Feuchtwang, Stephan. 2011. *After the Event: The Transmission of Grievous Loss in Germany, China and Taiwan*. New York: Berghahn Books.

Hirsch, Marianne. 2008. The Generation of Postmemory. *Poetics Today* 29 (1): 103–128.

Jing, Jun. 1996. *The Temple of Memories: History, Power, and Morality in a Chinese Village*. Stanford: Stanford University Press.

Lass, Andrew. 1994. From Memory to History. The Events of November 17 Dis/Remembered. In *Memory, History, and Opposition under State Socialism*, ed. Ruby Watson. Santa Fe: School of American Research Press.

Pickering, Michael, and Emily Keightley. 2013. Communities of Memory and the Problem of Transmission. *European Journal of Cultural Studies* 16 (1): 115–131.

Pine, Frances. 2007. Memories of Movement and Stillness of Place: Kinship Memory in the Polish Highlands. In *Ghosts of Memory: Essays on Remembrance and Relatedness*, ed. Janet Carsten. Oxford: Blackwell.

Renshaw, Layla. 2011. *Exhuming Loss: Memory, Materiality and Mass Graves of the Spanish Civil War*. Walnut Creek, CA: Left Coast.

Riesco, Sergio. 2006. La intensificación de cultivos durante la Reforma Agraria de la II República: ¿Alternativa o complemento?. In *¿Interés particular, bienestar público? Grandes patrimonios y reformas agrarias*, ed. Rîcardo Robledo, Hernández Santiago. M., and López García. Zaragoza: Universidad de Zaragoza Prensas de Zaragoza.

Rothberg, Michael. 2009. *Multidirectional Memory: Remembering the Holocaust in the Age of Decolonization*. Stanford: Stanford University Press.

Sánchez Marroyo, Fernando. 1990. Las Organizaciones Obreras en Extremadura durante la Segunda República. *Investigaciones históricas: época moderna y contemporánea* 10: 123–164.

Skultans, Vieda. 1998. *The Testimony of Lives: Narrative and Memory in Post-Soviet Latvia*. London and New York: Routledge.

Wagner, Sarah E. 2008. *To Know Where He Lies: DNA Technology and the Search for Srebrenica's Missing*. Berkeley, CA and London: University of California Press.

CHAPTER 6

The Affective Life of Violence

In the context of the exhumations of Castuera and Puebla de Alcocer, one could say that in order to understand the killings of those in the mass graves and the impact of those murders on people's lives and identities, one needs to transgress the space of the mass burial and follow the trail of these deaths into the stories of postwar repression and familial mourning that were articulated at each excavation site. In his famous work *The Order Has Been Carried Out*, Alessandro Portelli (2003) sets out to investigate the massacre of the Fosse Ardeatine in Rome, where Nazi forces killed over three hundred Italian prisoners, presumably in retaliation for each of the German soldiers who died as a result of a partisan bomb planted in via Rasella (Rome) in 1944. In the book, Portelli explains the need to contest the nature of this story as a "single, self-enclosed event" (ibid., 12). His purpose then becomes that of expanding the rigid boundaries—the fixed beginning and end—that the story of Fosse Ardeatine acquired in its different popular and official versions, in order to understand the event in connection to the broader spectrum of circumstances that surrounded both mass killings from a historical viewpoint. As in the case of Fosse Ardeatine, the story of the killings in Castuera and Puebla did not start and end with these men's executions. In both scenarios archival and oral narratives about the deaths hinted at a previous context to which the killings needed to be related, but also to a later time in which these stories and their repercussions remained latent in each locality.

Z. Aragüete-Toribio, *Producing History in Spanish Civil War Exhumations*, World Histories of Crime, Culture and Violence,
DOI 10.1007/978-3-319-61270-6_6

In the case of Castuera, the most immediate context was provided by the events surrounding the end of the war and the management of prisoners through the emerging military justice and detention system near the disintegrated front of Extremadura. In Puebla, the killings have to be understood in the context of the local confrontations where these *sacas* or executions took place—also at the end of the war. The encounter with the mass grave by those of later generations, especially the children of the defeated, prompted other types of vivid reminiscence, marked by the absence of these relatives in the family and by a history of starvation, poverty, discrimination, and presumed solidarity in Franco's Spain. Moreover, these experiences of familial absence provided a context for the traumatic historical search that many relatives have carried out in recent years and which, ultimately, gave a strong personal meaning to the exhumation practice. The accounts of families that could not find the bodies of their relatives in Castuera and the life histories shared in Puebla evidenced the haunting and affective afterlife (Gordon 1997; Navaro-Yashin 2012; Das 2007; Hirsch 2012) of these mass and individual killings in familial relations, in each village's social politics, and in the mournful experience of the relatives of the defeated over time, from the postwar to the moment of the exhumation and beyond.

The Trails of the Dead in Postwar Memories

For the archaeologists, the compilation of stories about the postwar period was again in line with the project's aim, and thus with Laura Muñoz Encinar's approach to the study of the mass grave: taken not in isolation but as an element that was part of the wider repressive Francoist apparatus, which extended into the postwar period. Stories of postwar repression shared at both sites blurred the established ending that the event received in many narratives—among them, those from Francoist historians—which have presented these killings as an occurrence that did not transcend the war. The harsh reality of the postwar period, however, was a widely cited issue in the accounts provided by many family members I interviewed. Conversing with relatives made one aware of the difficulties most had in describing how their kin had been killed. As Chaps. 4 and 5 have shown, most of the narratives from the direct descendants of those who disappeared or were executed evidenced how time, secrecy, and fear around the telling of these events had dispersed details about these brutal deaths over generations. In contrast, the subject of the postwar period was vividly invoked as a moment of extreme suffering and endurance, whose experience was crucial in the shaping of the subjectivities of those who survived.

Certainly, during interviews, people would prefer to draw from personal stories, which delved into the quotidian character of the postwar period, associating hardship with the absence of their dead kin and the decrepit conditions in which the war left their households. These narratives emphasized the effects of war violence, especially disappearance and death, over these families' futures. They elucidated the way in which the living, as Veena Das (1996, 88) has pointed out about the lives of sexually abused women in India, "build a world that he or she can inhabit" in the aftermath of violence. In a situation in which neighbours who had supported the legitimacy of the Second Republic had to coexist with those who backed the uprising and Francoist regime after the conflict, people's everyday lives became marked by the onerous nature of these relations and the pressure exerted over the lives of those connected to the Republican past. Violence, recalling Das (2007) again, descended into their ordinary lives, leading to decades of hardship. According to many accounts, in such conditions life became more strenuous and unbearable than death when the conflict ended. This, as the great-granddaughter of a woman who was imprisoned for 14 years explained to me in Puebla de Alcocer, was especially the case for women in Puebla, for most of those killed in the village were men. As Luisa Cabanillas Bayón, a 74 years old woman, also from Puebla, whose father was killed and mother sentenced to 30 years and a day in prison after the war, explained in an interview:

> My mother used to say: "the years I spent with your father were the happiest." She could not feed us, five girls, sometimes… When she was released from jail, I heard her say on more than one occasion: "How comfortably you rest Luis, you got two shots and everything ended for you, but I…" (Luisa Cabanillas Bayón, Puebla, August 2012)

The words of Luisa's mother resonated with the postwar experience of many other families I met in Puebla and elsewhere in Extremadura.[1] Portelli (2003, 9) has also stressed the role that women have played "in surviving and remembering" experiences such as the massacre of the Fosse Ardeatine. In Puebla and Castuera, women's narratives retold the history of a struggle for continuity in which the reforming mission of the Francoist authorities politically contained the lives of these widows and their offspring in the public realm. Luisa's story, for instance, was representative of the punishment that some wives and daughters of socialist men killed at the end of the conflict underwent in different prisons around the country. Luisa's mother, Presentación Bayón Villarejo, had been married to Luis Cabanillas Herrera, who was trialled by court-martial and killed in Badajoz in 1940. Presenta, as people knew her, was arrested in 1939 and jailed with her sister Dolores, Luis's sister Agustina—Pablo Trenado's mother—and other fellow female neighbours, first in Puebla and later, after their military trial, in other prisons in cities like Durango and Saturrarán (Basque Country). As happened to many women, Presenta learnt about her husband's execution in prison. As an infant, Luisa grew up with Presenta in prison, staying with her until she was four years old. Her cousin Pepa was also with her aunt Agustina. When Luisa visited the exhumation site she still remembered those years vividly and even sang, next to the mass grave, at the moment of the exhumation, the songs of longing the inmates used to intone in Durango and Saturrarán. She recalled living in prison and going to the prison school, which was run by nuns, the poor conditions and malnutrition inmates sustained, and the threat of being given to another family for adoption—her cousin Pepa was nearly taken away, she remembered, as nuns tried to convinced Pepa's mother she would be happier with a more affluent family in the Basque Country. Agustina was eventually released after four years, and Presenta was released after she completed the first eight years of her thirty-year sentence. The girls were sent back home earlier. Images of the prison never escaped Luisa's memory, who still remembered its rooms and corridors, the bedside table where her mother kept her father's letters, and the bridge they crossed to reach the sea.

When Luisa spoke about her own return to Puebla without her mother, aged four, she summoned the image of her poverty-stricken family. Whilst their mother was in jail, her grandmother and two of her aunts looked after Luisa and her four sisters. From an early age, she remembered strongly the image of two of her sisters, who lived with one of her aunts were barefoot and only wearing a shirt, weakened by the famine that devastated the family: "if they were sent to the fountain to get water, they couldn't: they fell because they could not walk!" In the postwar-related stories people told, hunger was a recurrent theme and temporal marker—stories often recalled the "years of famine",

1941 being the most taxing moment—which brought out information about the conditions in which the war left the region and the subsistence economy that gradually emerged in Puebla and other villages. Reflecting on time and subjectivity in *Life and Words*, Veena Das (2007, 95–107) discusses how people's narratives of suffering reveal a perception of time that is enmeshed with their personal experience of collective and individual violence. This phenomenal time, which ultimately defines the affective qualities of past events in the present, often brings specific moments into sharp relief whilst portraying broader accounts of daily struggle. The reference to hunger in Puebla, then, should be understood as a continuing experience, which marked people's lives and was deeply entangled with other forms of poverty, exclusion, expropriation and inequality that deeply affected Republicans—"widows, orphans, those exiled and the victims of repression and their families" (Agustí and Mir 2005, 75).

Many authors have attributed the dramatic situation in the country in those years to the lack of provisions (Molinero and Ysás 2003; Agustí et al. 2005). Some have observed that the depuration of many workers considered hostile to the regime during the war, their dismissal for previous affiliations in the postwar period, or the extreme salary reductions during the instauration of the Francoist regime led to the "extraordinary deterioration of wage earner's daily lives [...] in a climate of general dearth" (Molinero and Ysás 2003). José's father, for instance, remembered working just for food during those years of famine. Moreover, the regime's rationing system, approved in 1939, was highly deficient, giving place to a soon-established and long-lasting black market (ibid.). Molinero and Ysás (2003, 17) have further argued that the New Regime chose to enforce these supply policies in line with its autarkic project, which also enabled it to gain social control over the population. In Puebla, José Sánchez-Paniagua's mother-in-law, who often visited the exhumation, explained how she remembered begging, shoeless, for food on people's doorsteps when she was still an infant. This experience has also been recalled by Ángel Sayabera in Castuera, when, after his parents and brothers disappeared, he begged with his blind grandfather. Everyone I interviewed spoke about how people went to the grazing lands and valleys located next to villages to pick up thistle, which was then peeled and cooked in water, or how others ate fried potato peels. On many occasions, people uttered their pain through these stories of scarcity and hunger, making the past feel very present (Das 2007).

For many, these circumstances were aggravated, as some have observed (Renshaw 2011), by the looting and theft of belongings and property of Republican families at the end of the war. These forms of expropriation that many identified in their accounts had been firstly informally carried out and later legislated through the *Ley de Responsabilidades Políticas* (Law of Political Responsibilities), as punishment for their "political crimes" (Renshaw 2011, 99). In Castuera, Maria Hormeño and Aurora Navas recalled how their families' houses were seized and confiscated, retelling how fellow residents of the village had taken and distributed their possessions amongst a few. As pointed out also by other life histories, Maria remembered seeing her family's clothes and furniture in other people's houses. In our interview, she remembered how people could not usually claim these items back, though her mother, with the help of a neighbour from a well-to-do family, managed to recuperate her double bed, owned by a man who had acquired it after its expropriation. According to her, when her mother went to reclaim the item a second time—after the man had refused to give it to her on the first occasion—she told him that, if he did not like to own things that belonged to "reds," he should hand the bed back to her, for she was one. Talking about the loss of these material possessions was also a way of articulating the complex negotiation of one's previous being and identity in the new political milieu. Her mother's desperation and sense of urgency in recovering the bed for her household, where five members of the family shared one bed, prompted this moment of political labelling and differentiation. Nonetheless, Maria also recalled the impossibility of claiming other belongings imbued with memories of a pre-war lifetime, when as a young adult she walked on the street where her old house stood, and looked at, it regretting:

> I was born there and lived there for three or four years, my parents got married in that house [...] You could not say that. (Maria Hormeño, Castuera, 2011)

In the stories of second and third generations these episodes of *miseria* (misery)—as people often referred to them—also mixed with expressions of aid and cooperation among some neighbours, as Maria's case suggests. In Puebla, when grandchildren from third generations like Begoña and

Jacinto Velasco reflected on their grandmother's life without their grandfather Pelayo, they remarked how the memories they had were associated with her continuous "battle for survival". Begoña explained that in the first years after the conflict, their family, as many others, sought shelter in some of their closest neighbours, especially those who lived on the same street and were in a similar situation. Since they did not have much to share, Begoña added, "they fed their spirit rather than their hunger" (Begoña Velasco, Puebla, 2012). The story of Begoña's grandmother invoked reciprocity gestures through the lack of goods and food, uniting some in the community around their experiences of dearth. Other stories, however, described the development of informal networks of favours and exchanges among neighbours, embedded in the asymmetry of the social relations that emerged between victors and the defeated after the war.

In Puebla and Castuera, seemingly selfless acts of patronage and other forms of social advocacy co-habited in the social realm with state practices that aimed to alleviate the effects of poverty and starvation. In connection to this institutional aid, many authors have discussed how new forms of social assistance that emerged as a consequence of an economic project—backed by the State and the Church (i.e., *Auxilio Social* and *Acción Católica*)—tapped into these collectives, providing help but also demanding an ideological commitment to Franco's national-syndicalist (Giménez Muñoz 2009) and national-Catholic blueprint and its "re-Christianizing activity" (Montero García 2005, 117). Other types of aid, as some historians like Julián Chaves (2005) have observed, such as the so-called *socorros* or limited maintenance subsidies given to prisoners throughout the war were used, at some points, as propaganda to prove the benevolence of the New Regime towards the defeated. The documents shown below, compiled during José Sánchez-Paniagua's research into Puebla's municipal archive, exemplify these forms of institutionalized assistance given by the Civil Government of the province to those arrested in the village. The list includes neighbours' names—among them Agustina and Luis Cabanillas Herrera, Luisa's father and aunt—and an amount in old *pesetas* next to each person's details for collection. The back of the document shows the signatures of those listed, who collected their contribution (Fig. 6.1).

Narratives of survivors also retold informal exchanges that took place between neighbours at local level since the end of the conflict. In the postwar period, according to some accounts, it was mostly those

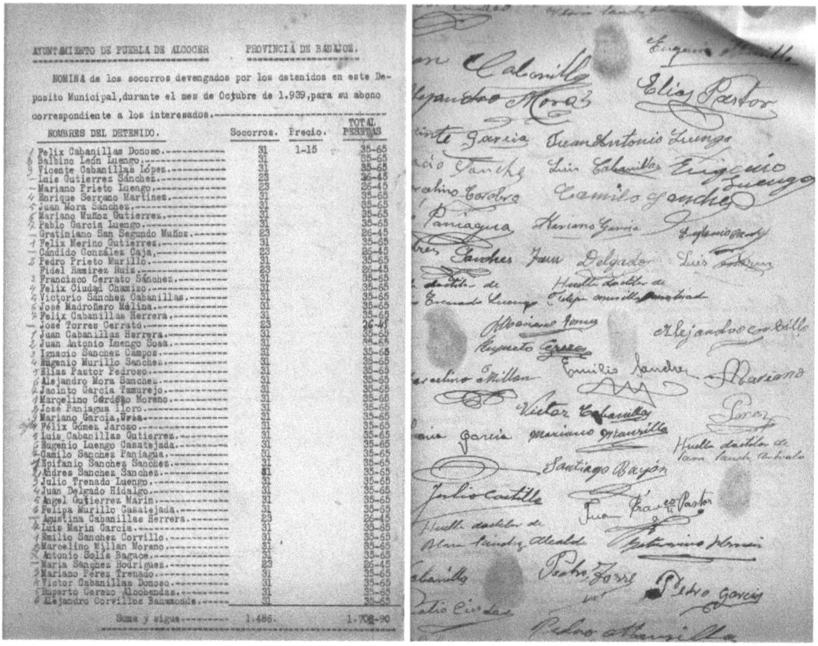

AYUNTAMIENTO DE PUEBLA DE ALCOCER PROVINCIA DE BADAJOZ.

NOMINA de los socorros devengados por los detenidos en este Deposito Municipal, durante el mes de Octubre de 1.939, para su abono correspondiente a los interesados.

NOMBRES DEL DETENIDO.	Socorros.	Precio.	TOTAL PESETAS
Felix Cabanillas Donoso.	31	1-15	35-65
Balbino León Luengo.	31		35-65
Vicente Cabanillas López.	31		35-65
Luis Gutierrez Sánchez.	23		26-45
Mariano Prieto Luengo.	23		26-45
Enrique Serrano Martinez.	31		35-65
Juan Mora Sánchez.	31		35-65
Mariano Muñoz Gutierrez.	31		35-65
Pablo García Luengo.	31		35-65
Gratiniano San Segundo Muñoz.	23		26-45
Felix Merino Gutierrez.	31		35-65
Cándido Gonzáles Caja.	23		26-45
Pedro Prieto Murillo.	31		35-65
Fidel Ramirez Ruiz.	23		26-45
Francisco Cerrato Sánchez.	31		35-65
Felix Ciudad Chamizo.	31		35-65
Victorio Sánchez Cabanillas.	31		35-65
José Madroñero Málina.	31		35-65
Felix Cabanillas Herrera.	31		35-65
José Torres Cerrato.	23		26-45
Juan Cabanillas Herrera.	31		35-65
Juan Antonio Luengo Sosa.	31		35-65
Ignacio Sanchez Campos.	31		35-65
Eugenio Murillo Sanchez.	31		35-65
Elias Pastor Pedroso.	31		35-65
Alejandro Mora Sanchez.	31		35-65
Jacinto García Tamurejo.	31		35-65
Marcelino Cárdeño Moreno.	31		35-65
José Paniagua Iloro.	31		35-65
Mariano García, Uría.	31		35-65
Félix Gómez Jarozo.	31		35-65
Luis Cabanillas Gutierrez.	31		35-65
Eugenio Luengo Casatejada.	31		35-65
Camilo Sanchez Paniagua.	31		35-65
Epifanio Sanchez Sanchez.	31		35-65
Andres Sanchez Sanchez.	31		35-65
Julio Trenado Luengo.	31		35-65
Juan Delgado Hidalgo.	31		35-65
Angel Gutierrez Marin.	31		35-65
Felipa Murillo Casatejada.	31		35-65
Agustina Cabanillas Herrera.	23		26-45
Luis Marin García.	31		35-65
Emilio Sanchez Corvillo.	31		35-65
Marcelino Millan Moreno.	31		35-65
Antonio Solís Bagace.	31		35-65
Maria Sanchez Rodriguez.	23		26-45
Mariano Perez Trenado.	31		35-65
Victor Cabanillas Donoso.	31		35-65
Ruperto Cerezo Alcobendas.	31		35-65
Alejandro Corvillos Banamonde.	31		35-65
Suma y sigue	1.486.		1.708-90

Fig. 6.1 List of prisoners and *socorros* in Puebla de Alcocer and prisoners' receipt signatures. Courtesy of José Sánchez-Paniagua

well-to-do families considered to be right-wing, who could provide aid for the families of the defeated, and to prisoners too. For instance, at the end of the war, many prisoners secured their release through a written endorsement from someone trusted and well regarded by the new authorities in the village—usually from one of these wealthy families in agreement with the new order. Securing this endorsement was key to the release and for them to be able to return to their village of origin—as some, even if freed, were forced to go into exile in neighbouring cities or villages. In Puebla de Alcocer, Presenta, Luisa's mother, Agustina, and all those who went through jail—others like Emiliano had also been imprisoned in Castuera concentration camp at the end of the war—secured this endorsement from people who had been family friends in the past and aligned, after the war, with the winning side of the conflict. However, according to Luisa, this aid was often hindered by the power of others over the lives of Republican families. Luisa often recalled that her mother was the last of the women to be released from Saturrarán, as the endorsement for her acquittal was held in Puebla for years by the local head of Falange. These forms of civil endorsement or *avales* were mentioned in all stories of detention. *Avales* certified the trustworthiness of those considered the enemy, though in many cases—as happened to Ángel Sayabera's brother in Castuera, killed before his warrant reached him—local and prison authorities ignored them. The contrast between the acts of cooperation between some families and those influenced by the intentions of Francoist authorities and neighbours were always at odds in the subjective experience narrated by those members of the left-wing families who survived. Relationships between neighbours, as in other contexts (Das 2007; Sanford 2003), were constantly negotiated around the communities' public secrets: the past atrocities committed, betrayals, and ongoing forms of postwar violence and coercion in the community.

When Presenta returned home, Luisa remembered, she had nothing. The same people who secured her discharge also offered her some land on lease to grow cereals. She lived with Luisa's grandmother and recovered her five daughters whilst she worked her wheat field, made bread, and sold it on the black market (*estraperlo*). Many women I interviewed, who were in the same situation, were eventually given work by some of the village's wealthiest families or by neighbours within the new regime. Many even worked for those who had denounced their relatives early on. Others, like Aurora Navas's aunt in Castuera, with whom she grew up, married members from Falange or right-wing men who helped them in the postwar period and provided an education for their children. Moreover, in numerous cases documented in Puebla, working in life-long positions as maids or as property guards in the countryside, in the case of men, became commonplace. José and Consuelo's grandmother, for instance, worked as a maid for a Francoist teacher called Doña Nati almost until the end of her life. The teacher was recalled in numerous stories for the help she gave to families of socialist neighbours killed at the end of the war.

Esperanza Muga also fondly remembered the figure of Doña Nati, as she became a friend when many discriminated against the family for their political past. In Esperanza's account, Doña Nati's aid was significant, especially after her mother and uncle were arrested on suspicion of collaborating with the anti-Francoist guerrilla gathered in the nearby mountains, known in the village as *los de la sierra* (*maquis* or people on the mountains). Allegedly, it was someone from the community who falsely accused and reported them to the police, in an act of rancour. Both mother and uncle spent months in prison. According to Francisco Cobo Romero (2005, 42) the denunciation—or *delación*—of "the enemy or unwanted neighbour" was promoted as a form of civil collaboration with the new authorities. It became common practice, which, as the author highlights, was often moved by pre-war controversies and articulated through trivial accusations (ibid.). After Eperanza's mother and uncle were taken away, she and her brother stayed with their grandmother, for she was their only relative alive and out of prison. Doña Nati assisted the family and alleviated the children's loss, especially since in the ensuing months the family experienced ongoing harassment from the local Civil Guard after their relatives were detained. Their menacing treatment marked Esperanza's perception of the postwar years:

> At night, the three of us slept on the same bed because we were so scared. I slept with my grandmother on the upper part of the bed whilst my brother slept at the bottom. In the middle of the night, they came banging on the door to make us even more frightened. My grandmother said 'shhh', so we remained quiet. They banged on the door at night with very loud thwacks… they just wanted to make us all scared! (Esperanza Muga, Puebla, 2012)

Certainly some people connected some of these charitable acts described to me to the kindness and solidarity of the person who performed them. Others seemed to me to be embedded in the emerging humanitarian expressions of the New Regime that aimed to consolidate its salvation rhetoric. In reminiscing about this postwar reality, humanitarian narratives were mixed with vigorous descriptions of the coercion many endured from other neighbours. Postwar stories of fear, depravation, and familial suffering that many life histories such as Esperanza's depicted gave other meanings to the deaths of the men in the mass graves, verbalizing the haunting force of their absence (Das 2007). In Puebla de Alcocer and Castuera these stories, retold at the excavation site and in people's houses, conjured the affective memory of the dead in these village communities during the dictatorship and pointed to the effect of their absent presence on social politics and familial distress. Moreover, the voices of those who experienced the agony and ubiquitous insecurity of the postwar period, found, in the arena of the exhumation, a space from which to finally denounce the identity of those who perpetrated the crimes.

As opposed to other studies such as Renshaw's (2011), which shows how second and third generations never addressed the names of perpetrators at one of the mass graves the author analyses, in contexts such as Puebla (more than in Castuera), for instance, these names occupied the same space as those of the men executed, with survivors' or those of the neighbours who provided help to left-wing families after the war. The exhumation site provided a certain sense of intimacy in which a form of accountability could be uttered. In Puebla, on repeated occasions, these narratives spoke about the neighbours and military men who accompanied the prisoners to the trenches when they were going to be killed and their behaviour in the aftermath. Many neighbours recounted how, upon returning to the village, the perpetrators celebrated the murders, evoking the popular ritual of the "pig killing"—or *matanza*[2]—whilst they drank and ate in one of the village's bars. Often when recalled, perpetrators were remembered for their role in community affairs, for their wrongdoings, and for the way they died. In these cases, their deaths were explained as if their lurid endings had followed from the bad deeds they committed. For instance, in Puebla, many talked about how one of these men died when a bolt of lightning hit him as he walked around during the annual livestock *fiesta*. In such a way, the lives and fates of victims and perpetrators were continually woven, composing a vision of social contention and its impact on familial and individual existence over time.

Other stories also recounted different forms of persecution, surveillance, and punishment during the postwar years, involving the police, the Civil Guard, and the local authorities. For instance, many endured the constant vigilance of the regime's authorities, though some were oblivious to it. The police and authorities, for instance, monitored Luisa's mother, after she was released from jail, for the entire duration of her original thirty-year prison sentence. Her family, however, only learnt this later on, realizing her sentence had come to an end, in 1969—three years after Presenta had passed away. For most surviving relatives, the adversity they underwent prompted them to leave their home villages and migrate to other cities in the country, partly because of the poverty that overcame these rural areas and due to the stigma bestowed upon them by the political past with which they were associated. In the case of Maria Hormeño in Castuera, she left the village when she was an adolescent and never came back to live there again. In our interview, she expressed on several occasions how the arduous reality of village life triggered her departure, explaining how she only came back to see the family she left behind. In other cases, many stories told by second and third generation relatives at the exhumation site emphasized the positive treatment that their relatives and families had enjoyed in the village and the fondness they felt for the town. When these experiences were recounted, they starkly contrasted the descriptions that many official files and propaganda conveyed of their Republican ancestors. Many stories willingly or unwittingly reasserted the goodness and integrity of the widows, children, and grandchildren of the defeated, resisting and contesting other Francoist visions. Stories such as Luisa's at the end of the piece point to the esteem and love that defined her relationship with others in Puebla's community, for her mother never "passed rancour" onto her offspring. As Luisa further explained to me in an interview:

> This village, Puebla the Alcocer, was formed by landowners and then all the poor. I worked for all of them [landowners] and I got along with all of them, but many of them knew what they had done. Nonetheless, every one of them treated my mother really well... if you ask anyone in the village about my mother they would say: 'Presenta, the best woman there is...'. (Luisa Cabanillas Bayón, Puebla, 2012)

Experiences such as Luisa's and Maria's draw out the "burdens and tensions" (Portelli 2003, 13) of the postwar milieu and how the unrealized mourning of those left alive shaped their experience and that of later generations. Postwar stories told by the gravesite and elsewhere evinced how "singular individuals inscribed themselves in a [social] history" (Miñarro and Morandi 2013, 22). Theirs and other stories helped me to discern during fieldwork, as other authors have recognized (Miñarro and Morandi 2013), how guilt, untold pain and shame articulated subjective feelings during the postwar period, forging a culture of trauma, which imbued the relation between survivors, descendants and their communities. Such an underlying grief determined the memory-work of different generations. In more recent years, it has also structured the process of information collection on the part of the children and grandchildren of the defeated about their familial histories. For descendants, the information in archives and oral accounts—and later at the exhumation—embodied the suffering of the dead and the traces of a past not fully fathomed or completed. In their inquiry, their experiences of familial transmission shaped the assemblage of personal biographical narratives, in which ancestors' stories were written and such suffering confronted. These acts of searching and writing performed by some relatives were thus suffused with an unrelenting desire to place the defeated, and also themselves, in history.

Writing a History of Trauma

Throughout the time I spent in Extremadura in 2011 and 2012, interviews and informal conversations, especially with second- and third-generation descendants of those who lived the violence of the war, unveiled the different ways in which the past had reached them as part of familial exchanges. Some psychoanalytical studies such as Miñarro and Morandi (2013) have argued that knowledge transmission is essential in the formation of identities within the family nucleus. These authors discuss, inspired by Freud, how transmission in filial relations "operates through identification" (ibid., 83). Within the family, such processes of identification, which create affective links between its members, are based on the unconscious appropriation of parental attitudes, behaviours, or emotional traits. In the case of the transmission of traumatic experiences, these authors observe that a lack of words or narratives about the disturbing events of the war gave way to the unconscious appropriation by children of parental pain and suffering.

Many stories I heard retold the way in which parents' distress travelled between generations, impregnating family bonds and making an imprint on children and grandchildren's feelings and knowledge about the past. A man who I met at a commemorative act in Castuera, for instance, once told me that he could feel his father's affliction—caused by his experience as a prisoner in different concentration Camps and later in forced labour battalions around the country—because he vividly recalled the endless bitterness (*estaba siempre amargao*) that filled the house when he returned home from his imprisonment. Similarly, at a different commemorative event, another woman recounted to me how distress about the past had always been marked by the times when she asked her father about the war and he, unable to speak about it, closed his fists in anger until he made his hands bleed (*cerraba los puños con fuerza hasta que le sangraban*). People's accounts often pointed to the effects of a perpetuated silence, as well as the explicit ways in which some sentiments were manifested—not only through fragmented narratives but also through gestures and actions that impressed everyday routines.

Trauma moved through transgenerational forms of affective transmission, toying with secrecy and spreading through different genealogies (Cho 2008). In some cases, words would be articulated in incomprehensible parts. In others, expressions of sadness and despair would manifest, as above, through the enactment of pain in a quietened familial space of transmission. This deadened space, in which transmission was hard to articulate and suffering never explicitly uttered, was transformed when many relatives of the defeated began to compile files, stories, images, and writings about their ancestors' war and postwar experiences to create personal archives and produce narratives about their life histories. These activities of collection and recollection were directly entwined with the uncertainty that surrounded their kin's past and with the impossibility of placing their own lives in a historical continuum. As Marianne Hirsch (2012, 31) has remarked about the search for the past in post-Holocaust generations, these acts and objects are part of "transactive and transferential processes" that not only "transform history into memory, but enable memories to be shared across individuals and generations." The memory that results from these elaborations, Hirsch argues, are not identical to those from the first generations of survivors, though they resemble "their affective force and its physical effects" (ibid.).

This historical quest opened other avenues for the experience of a dislodged trauma, as the new information found was enmeshed with the politics of the official archive and the anxieties trapped in the accounts of the war and postwar period, in which the trails of the dead and his or her absence survived. As in the case witnessed in Chap. 3, where the documents that certified the death of José González Barrero disturbed his daughter Libertad due to the inauthentic details found in them about his killing, the process of information gathering carried out by those families that frequented the exhumations in Castuera and Puebla de Alcocer revealed the affective capacity of these sources in the transformation of relatives' experience of the past. Considering these personal searches into their familial pasts involves the retracing of how and when these stories *returned* to their everyday or how the story of disappearance or death came to be owned by later generations again after a long period of silence. The process of recollection these relatives embarked upon is undoubtedly linked to what Cathy Caruth (1995, 1996) has termed the historical power of trauma. Forged through the latency and abeyance of disturbing or tragic events—in the stillness and cracks of postwar remembrance—a sense of lived and inherited trauma propelled the pursuit and accumulation of clues about a perceived yet unknown troublesome past. In this context, and as the author argues, trauma becomes not so much a symptom of the mind in the aftermath of a distressful occurrence but of history itself, as its belatedness made its experience only possible in relation to "another place and another time" (Caruth 1995, 8).

For the relatives I met in Castuera, for whom the disappearance and death of their kin had been filled with so much perplexity from the start, the assemblage of information threw light on a blurry familial reality and its place in the society of the time. Just as for the children of Holocaust survivors discussed by Hirsch (2012), it unlocked a process of constant re-imagination of an uncertain past through testimonies and archival materials. In the case of Maria Hormeño's daughter Marielo Gil Hormeño, discovering new information about the past of her mother's family, as she compellingly described, was "like, suddenly, finding a room in your house you had never seen before" (Marielo Gil Hormeño, Castuera, 2011). In an interview, Marielo explained how throughout her life she had pieced the story of her grandfather, Antonio Hormeño, through the scattered information she had received from her mother when growing up and from the stories she heard as a young adult. Marielo observed that when chatting to her mother the stories she told about her father's disappearance and the events that preceded it were never linear. The atmosphere in the house, she pointed out, was never apt for the telling of some stories, as the widespread silence over these events during the dictatorship, but also the fact that her father was, in her words, "a very right-wing man," conditioned her mother's disposition to speak.

Later on in her life, Marielo started working on a family tree. Her research there would confront her with the serendipitous reality of her mother's family story, which comprised not only the killing of her grandfather but also of three of her grandfather's brothers. After requesting information from civil registries about her relatives' deaths, she learnt that out of the seven brothers registered in her mother's family only some had death certificates. These "anomalies," as she referred to them, made her abandon the idea of the family tree and instead concentrate on a search for information about the relatives who disappeared at the end of the conflict. It was through Marielo's research that the memory of her absent kin returned to conversations held between her and her mother Maria. Her adamant interest led her to contact different historians around the country and in Extremadura through internet forums and sites where names and details about those who were killed and disappeared are shared between researchers and families. In our interview, she vividly remembered the moment when she found a historian who held information about one of Maria's disappeared uncles, José Hormeño—who was allegedly Castuera town mayor from 1937—and what she felt when, at the same time, she realized that, after much searching, no information remained about her grandfather's death:

> When I started researching, I didn't know where to start. I hardly knew anything about the Civil War. I only had a general knowledge of it. Then, the internet became everything. I searched and found a historians' forum. In a similar way as when you throw a coin into the air, I sent an email to the list asking: 'Does anyone know José Hormeño?' I thought no one would answer. It feels unbelievable to me now… The next day when I opened my email I had a message that read: 'I have information about José Hormeño.' I looked at the subject of the email for a minute, without having the courage to open it. I felt so emotional that I didn't dare to open it. When I finally did, this man tells me that he is a historian writing a book at the time called the *Column of Death [La Columna de la Muerte]* and that in his files the name of José Hormeño appeared together with that of his brothers… I wrote back to him and he provided me with information about where they had been imprisoned, their military death sentences… He gave me the dates when they were executed and where they were buried and again, I encountered the disappointing reality that there [was] no information about the whereabouts of my grandfather." (Marielo Gil Hormeño, Castuera, 2011)

The historian who provided her with these documents was Francisco Espinosa Maestre, a researcher who has broadly written about the development of the war in the province of Badajoz. When Marielo read the historian's message aloud to her mother, she said Maria "burst into tears as if her uncles had been killed that very moment" (Marielo Gil Ormeño, Castuera, 2011). Maria had never known details about the trial or executions of her uncles in the towns of Mérida and Almendralejo. She had encountered these unfamiliar events for the first time, after listening to the information extracted from the official archive that the historian had provided her daughter. Such an archival retrieval created a dreadful image of their execution never envisaged before through the pronouncements of their trial files. With the documents that the historian had passed on to Marielo, she was then able to further structure the family's story and ask her mother concrete questions about those aspects that remained doubtful. Public images and narratives of the official files became, through the work of the historian, mediators of "intimate familial transmission" (Hirsch 2012, 30).

Many of these documents stood in stark contrast to her mother's testimony and to other files that the historian Antonio López from Castuera provided her—such as the *avales* or endorsements her uncle José Hormeño received, whilst in jail, from right-wing neighbours he had saved from imprisonment and death during his time as town mayor at the beginning of the war. The documents from her uncles' court-martials and their sentences had, according to Marielo—and as Candela Chaves, the researcher from PREMHEx, once warned me—to be carefully examined. When Marielo spoke about the papers recovered from José Hormeño's trial, for instance, there was apprehension in her description of the information they contained. The accusations that the document comprised, she assured me, were general and customary, as shown in other court-martial sentences she had been able to review. Among other crimes, many people like her uncle were accused of "military rebellion," which to her made his indictment tenuous and premeditated. For Marielo, his accusation was highly representative of the aberrant character of these procedures and their equivocal nature. In his trial, she added, the public prosecutor rejected the civil endorsements presented by his defence, obliterating any chance of his being acquitted. For Maria's daughter, these processes were a "farce," which made the reading of these papers ultimately, in her words, "depressing."

Such documents helped, as Carolyn Steedman (2008) has argued evoking Ricoeur, to narrativize "absence into presence, and into time" in familial chronicles, just as historians materialised their information as part of a concrete social context and chronology. Their fraudulent kind triggered an analysis in conjunction with other sources, as Marielo's conversations with her mother elucidate, and also in relation to other materials present in the insidious archive. In their contact with archival sources, some families learnt to discern the language of the dictatorial regime and the contradictions held within its pages. Nonetheless, their search and their reading were challenging and unsettling. Just as the fever in the archive, in Derrida's terms, manifested itself in the exploration of files—but also in the practice of searching, attending, and living in the archive—for the professional historian (Steedman 2001), the quests initiated by these families led them to develop a similar relation to the source, in which such *mal d'archive* (Derrida 1996) was magnified through the effects of their personal grief. Entering the imagined space of the official archive and confronting its authority required an ability to figure out and decode Francoist commandments but also a strong will to face them. These documents had come into family's archives, like Maria and Marielo's, shaping a new historical consciousness and a retelling of familial stories of loss.

In the case of Ángel Sayabera in Castuera, for instance, files that documented the death certificates of his mother, father, and two brothers, whose deaths were inscribed in 1943, and which stated they died as a result of a "*clash against the public force*," coexisted with the array of additional documentation he had collected and written over the years. During our interview, Ángel spoke about the documents: he led us through the files of the civil registry provided by historian Antonio López; through his father's writing for the regional communist newspaper *Extremadura Roja* which he had recovered; through the last letter his father sent to his brother from Castuera concentration camp (see Chap. 4); and through the diversity of letters and pages Ángel himself had written (see Fig. 6.2). The latter formed a diary that recorded and retold the family's birth dates, details about their disappearances, and also the way they died. Other writings accounted for his present frustrations and demands for public acknowledgement of stories like his. Among Ángel's writings there were tales "to future generations" that aimed to tell, "the truth about what happened in the past"—as it was expressed in one of the documents. There were also letters addressed to local political representatives, such as the previous socialist town mayor in Castuera, and letters to the central government demanding the recognition of victims of Francoism. Ángel's compositions elicited his need to express himself, in his words, in a "space where one can talk again," provided by the recent historical memory movement. The intensive assortment and production of documents, in Ángel's case, resembles the infinite search of Sebald's Austerlitz for the traces of his mother. As Hirsch (2012, 44–45) describes, Sebald's character becomes fixated with a need to authenticate the presence of his mother at the concentration Camp of Terezín, where the Nazis deported her, only to encounter blurry and fuzzy images of her persona. Documents, images and other remnants provide for Ángel, as for Austerlitz, a space of "projection, approximation and affiliation," which has retained the aura of their relatives (ibid.).

Documents from the official archive travelled to the sphere of the domestic, where they interlaced with familial re-interpretations of their official narratives. Their content became part of a different private archive that aimed to evince the existence of relatives' disappeared

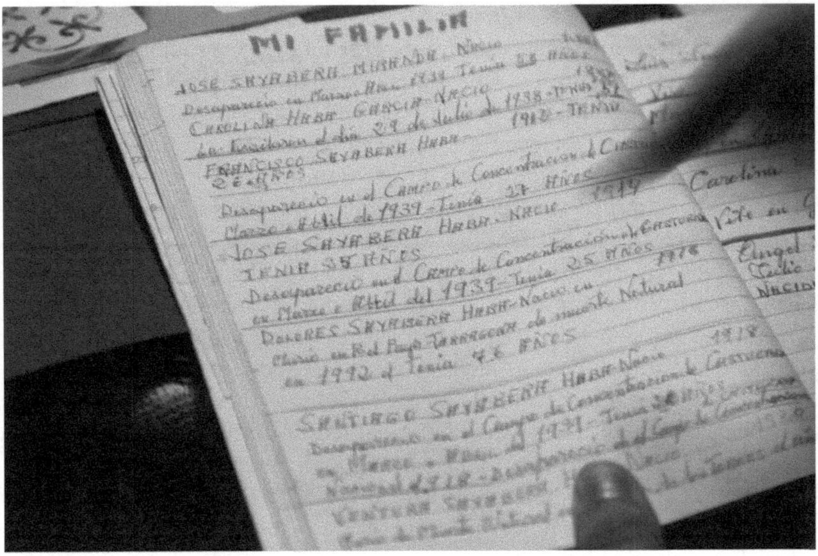

Fig. 6.2 Ángel's writing "Mi Familia" (My Family) where family birth and death dates are recorded, as well as causes of disappearance and death

ancestors and contest the uncertainty of the state files. In the case of Aurora Navas Morillo from Castuera, who only found out full details about her mother Matilde's death in 2002 ("until 2002 she was my great unknown", she said to me on one occasion), only three files remained with information about her kin in state repositories. Aurora had been able to locate, with the aid of historians and members of the administration, her birth and death certificate and Matilde's Teacher Purge File or *Expediente de Depuración*—with which she was dismissed from her position as a teacher in the town of Daimiel (Castilla La-Mancha). In an interview, Aurora explained to Laura Muñoz Encinar and I how the files she possessed clearly revealed, in her words, "the pantomime" of the administration at the time. When showing some of these documents to us, she carefully described the way in which her mother's death certificate and her Teacher Purge File—provided to her in this case by historian Julián Chaves Palacios—were fraught with discrepancies and contradicting indictments, making the search for information about her mother's fate futile and asserting her distrust in these sources.

The Teacher Purge File, signed on 7th April 1939, cleared Matilde and set her free from any charges. Upon returning to Castuera however, she was captured, incarcerated, and killed. Her deferred death certificate—made in 1946—establishes the date of her death on 30th March 1939, days before she had in fact signed her purge file in a different location. Against the perverse logic behind these antithetical inscriptions, other written papers and tokens in Aurora's collection constructed the trails of a counter-memory in her familial archive.

Examples of these counter-memories are the biographical notes Aurora read aloud for us at the beginning of the interview. In them Aurora had written the story of her father Antonio Navas, who had to go into exile due to his significant role in the socialist party (PSOE) and the trade union UGT. To craft her father's history, Aurora drew on files, provided by Antonio López, which included her father's correspondence with members of the party whilst in exile. In the story, she connected her mother to his life, creating a familial memory of Matilde as a mother, wife, and exemplary teacher. Just like Ángel, Aurora assured us that she wrote her father's biography for her grandchildren, so they could know who their great-grandfather and great-grandmother were. In such a way, the text stood as an emerging space for future transmission, elaborated in a third space, between the official archive and other familial remnants. In the absence of reliable documents about her mother's death, stories held in archival records would also stand in contrast with the memories and anecdotes shared in the inwardness of the home, where Aurora lived with her mother's sisters. The creation of these counter images, as anthropologists like Antoinette Burton (2003) have pointed out, turned the house into a space for history making throughout the years and in particular from the moment Aurora began her investigation into her mother's killing. The house was not only felt as a safe space to talk and intimately remember—especially after years of Francoist oppression—but also a space in which recollection could be crafted through the things that belonged to the deceased. In relation to the official file and their portrayal of Matilde's life and death, other objects and images in the house evoked her mother's presence and personality, thus confirming, in Aurora's words, that she *existed*. Her calligraphy books, the poems she read, and the images Aurora had managed to salvage helped her to construct a memory of her mother in which she believed and cherished. For Aurora, many of these things connected her to Matilde and her feelings, to the person she was. As she told us before reading aloud one of her mother's favourite poems by Heinrich Heine:

> I love reading this poem because my mother read it, because she also held the book like you and I are holding it now. There are so few things she touched that I can now touch. (Aurora Navas Morillo, Castuera, 2011)

Much of the writing, reading, and collecting with which families engage reclaims the memory of the deceased in an exercise of restoration—in conscious and unconscious ways. Much of the knowledge created in so doing relies not only on what is recorded or said in archives and oral narratives but also on the sensual and affective experience of these sources, on how they *feel*. The trail of those killed haunts the family archive, giving form to a reading of the past mutually constituted by the uncomfortable information in state files and involvement with other sources that evoke a trustworthy and emotive image of the deceased. The emotional engagement with the past generated through the research and recording of these stories determined contemporary representations of the defeated in familial but also social settings. In other cases, such intimate processes of collection and recollection transcended the realm of the family, making these explorations into the past part of a social project.

In Puebla de Alcocer, for instance, the research carried out by José Sánchez-Paniagua into the executions gave him motivation to assemble his family's story and create a compilation of the community's history. As already mentioned in Chap. 5, when José set out to investigate the killings, he aimed to discern, through the civil registry, the identities of all those buried with his grandfather. With time, however, his work led him to collect other documents, which spoke of the community as a whole and the intricate political and social relations that built it over time. Through the archive he discerned a myriad of events and fragments of particular life histories unknown to many families in the village. His research took him from his own family's past into the past of other neighbours. His contact with the archive also triggered an incessant search, moved by a personal desire to make Puebla's memory concrete. As he argued in our interview:

> This memory should never be forgotten, never. I am trying to learn all of Puebla's memory and I want to write about it… All of that memory will be read and seen and talked about. This is the most important thing. (José Sánchez-Paniagua, Puebla de Alcocer, 2012)

His research into Puebla's municipal archive helped him to deal with some of the uncertainties that the exhumation of the bodies presented—since through the archive, he trusted, he could identify the number of bodies found, which had not been accounted for at the start. The excavation, however, as seen in Chap. 5, also revealed for José the unreliability of the archival record in providing a faithful reading of the event of the killings. His experience, as he implied in one of our interviews, had showed him the importance of crosschecking, of comparing information with other historians' databases, and of "delving deeper into the archive" (José Sánchez-Paniagua, Puebla, 2012) to articulate a contrasted vision of the ambiguous aspects of Puebla's repressive past. Before and during the campaign José had been constant and mechanic in his treatment of the information, working with the diligent demeanour that I had observed in some of the historians I had interviewed before.

José firmly denied that he could be considered a "historian in the making" as I suggested to him, even if his developing skills in the archive and in collecting social histories presented a different reality. His extensive selection of carefully organized documents and recorded interviews, together with his writings about the exhumation and about some of the village stories on his online blog clearly reflected an emerging vocation that surpassed a mere new-found love for the craft of the historian. His work before, during, and after the excavation materialised his wish to articulate the town's history in an act of securing future recall. For José, historical consciousness was key to the village's existence, and he stressed that, "a village that forgets its history is doomed to disappear in the end" (José Sánchez-Paniagua, Puebla, 2012). His research was thus based on a vision of the continuity of the community through a collective awareness of the past. This will to foster the village's collective memory, also supported by the town hall, would later, after the exhumation, lead to the in-depth reconstruction of Puebla's municipal archive, destroyed in the wake of the war. José's work would then consist in the assemblage of the archival fund pre-1939, to throw light on the nineteenth and early-twentieth century in Puebla.

Puebla's social project, however, was not exempt from the predicaments caused by the violence contained in the archive. Delving into the municipal repository and reconstructing its afflictive pages would mark José's inner experience of the past and of the town in the present. The documents found by José in the humid cavities of Puebla's town hall were filled with familiar names and their sinuous and entangled stories of repression in the war and postwar-period village. As in the cases above, their content often triggered José's need to "constantly imagine what the person [on the document] underwent, their suffering…" especially when those examined spoke of his direct and distant relatives (José Sánchez-Paniagua, Puebla, 2012). José's research practice prompted the work of his individual imagination through the gruesome details he encountered. Much of the information about the repression in the village would transform his perception of the town as he knew it, its neighbours and spaces. Simultaneously, the historical flashes that unfolded through each document and image, when compiled, would unsettle his inherited memory.

For José, as for many of the families that embarked on research into their own histories, the making of such familiar and lineal narratives was filled with a frustration provoked by not knowing and exacerbated through the archive's "paltry truths," to evoke Ann Stoler's words (2009). The absence of the defeated and the reverberations of their deaths and disappearances lived in these processes of collection and recollection, as part of an unrelenting search fraught with grief. Through these acts of acquisition, accumulation, and interpretation the story of the defeated and the descendant were co-written. Such explorations into history created emerging representations of different familial pasts whilst shaping, conversely, the subjective worlds of those who engaged with them. The story of the dead and disappeared, as Portelli (2003) suggests in relation to Fosse Ardeatine, persisted and lingered through contained mourning and trapped emotions, marking the experience of the familial archive and, later, the day-to-day processes of the exhumation campaign.

Sentiment and Affect at the Exhumation Site

Previous chapters have discussed how knowledge about these killings was constructed at the excavation site, emphasizing the dialectics between local histories and scientific expertise. This knowledge, however, was also impregnated by the haunting trails of these deaths and the suffering they invoked—not only through the materiality registered in the mass grave but also the emotive stories of loss attached to it. The experiences of absence and adversity their presence recalled were part of the fabric of the exhumation space. They marked the perception of the site and its atmosphere, as well as the intimate relations people established with the mass grave and among themselves. The history concocted about the executions was hence also assembled through the sentiments and sensations produced in the interaction between the place, its materiality, and the subjective worlds that convened at the gravesite. The exhumation site, as well as the archive, was a harrowing space, in which the latent trauma that spread across generations overwhelmed the day-to-day of the excavation and the feelings that emerged in contact with it. Exhuming these human remains in Puebla de Alcocer and Castuera gained an intense and affective character for families and civil groups that promoted the historical memory project. It also deeply marked scientific practice and the intimate involvement of the archaeological team.

Anthropologist and archaeologist Leyla Renshaw (2011) has widely discussed the role of affect in Spanish Civil War exhumations, arguing how the mass grave becomes a space which profoundly affect those who come in touch with it. Among them, she focuses especially on the relations that scientists and volunteers establish with the mass grave arguing that they "do not simply facilitate these materializations [of the dead] through physical labour, or mediate representations of the past through experts readings; they are also profoundly affected by their encounters with their bodies and objects in the grave" (2011, 156). When I talk about affect, in this section, I mean, like Renshaw (ibid.) to refer to the capacity of these spaces, materialities, and stories to animate different behaviours in people and make them feel different things. Renshaw (2011) further describes, as I also appreciated during my field research, how the experience at the mass grave made many in the scientific team develop longer forms of political activism with projects and associations in Spain. Such contact with the open grave also made a powerful impact on their imagination, as they established novel personal relations with the corpses they excavated. In this context, however, one could say that bones are not just bones, or personal objects just any common item. They are part of the universe of these violent and personal histories and, as such, contain a strong emotive charge, which determines the intensities they irradiate.

Other definitions of affect, connect with what Yael Navaro-Yahin has called "complex affectivities" (Navaro-Yashin 2012, 134) in the context of the material remains of conflict that are left in northern Cyprus and whose presence concocts a particular experience of the post-violence Cypriot state and territory. Following Navaro-Yashin, I also speak about the affective potentialities of the space of the mass grave, produced by the desire and action of a new sovereign fascist power, and preserved as latent wounds that filled with discomfort and unease seemingly undisturbed landscapes. References to the executions and to the violence that took place were often invoked as participants of the exhumation

inhabited the space of the mass grave and listened to the stories of those who attended it over a prolonged period of time. There were also references to the victims' semblance and persona, to the perpetrators or the community in an effort to comprehend the event that marked each locality and which also had a strong impact on visitors, volunteers and archaeologists at the site. One could add to this, that it is again, through narrative and voice that such affective force became more poignant, as stories about the killings but also those which connected these to postwar absences in the household, entered the realm of the execution and mass burial ground.

For instance, on an occasion, after a day's work at the excavation site in Puebla de Alcocer, Lola, another archaeologist who worked with Laura in the direction of the campaign, reflected about her excavation experience in comparison to other sites at which she usually worked. Lola explained to me that in relation to the pre-historic sites to which she was accustomed, exhumations had an emotional load, which distressed the team and conditioned the dynamics of the work carried out. Indeed, she was not the first to acknowledge this. Previously another archaeologist, Álvaro, had stressed to me the sense of historical proximity these sites acquired through the familial and community narratives shared by the mass grave. For archaeologists, the excavation of these corpses often awakened feelings of unease, especially when the space was filled with war and postwar stories of families and survivors. Like Álvaro, Lola acknowledged how the act of retelling these disturbing events, together with the severe reality of the mass grave, impacted on the nature of the excavation. Nonetheless, her observations spoke further about how the exhumation affected the emotional responses of those who took part in it. In our conversation, Lola highlighted that one thing that astounded her was the profound capacity some of these stories had to stir all members of the team and even bring them all to tears. Lola expressed something we had all experienced in this and previous exhumations, especially when the space and the corpses were enveloped by the histories of direct relatives of the dead.

When José Sánchez-Panigua's father, José, came for the first time to the mass grave, silence overcame the excavation ground as he uttered his hope of being reunited with the human remains of his father. It was not only the harsh details of his detention and execution or what José recalled from his father's life history that moved those present at the site, but the flaring pain that erupted as he approached the excavation ground. Throughout the telling of his testimony, outbursts of tears and lament overcame his body, giving in to a tangle of nerves and shivers, triggered by his encounter with the corpses. Moments like this were difficult to negotiate in- and outside of the excavation ground. Such surging bodily expressions were the materialization of a lurking grief, which mixed with the uneasy sight of the corpses and defined the texture and feel of the space of the exhumation. For many members of the team, as I recorded on my field notes, the mass grave was at times a "sad place" from which an "uncomfortable energy" emanated.

Enmeshed with the landscape in which some of these stories were set, in the remoteness of the countryside in Puebla de Alcocer or connected to the moorlands of the concentration Camp in Castuera, the experience of these exhumation spaces was marked by the ill-fated aura they exuded. In Castuera, likewise, stories of prolonged disappearances and their repercussions on people's lives determined volunteers' engagement with familial emotions and the careful treatment of some of the information conveyed about the mass graves. In most cases, it was Laura Muñoz Encinar who communicated the initial hypotheses about the progress of the excavation, in an effort to avoid any ambiguity over the identity of the bodies in the graves. Though the archaeologist tried to maintain a distance with relatives' stories during the exhumation, for the impact their content could have on her work, Laura did deal with the hopes and uncertainties of families and activists on a daily basis, negotiating the meanings of the mass grave and the emotive responses of those involved in the campaign.

Away from the image of the exhumation as a dehumanized process, in which the body is simply turned into an "object of study" for scientific analysis, as some media discourses portray it (Domanska 2005), these exchanges with families displayed the most subjective side of scientific work in mass grave excavations (Renshaw 2011). The intimacy of the mass grave was also another realm in which transmission was performed and where affective materialities and memories challenged the sensibility of the researcher and volunteer. At the exhumation site, at times, members of the team assimilated themselves with the suffering contained in these histories of loss, in the form of storytelling, where the close sight and touch of these human remains triggered their imagination. The haunting effect of the dead encouraged an affinity and identification with such familial affliction, generating other anxieties in connection with their excavation practice.

Maria, one of the volunteers in Puebla, for instance, explained to me that experiencing the reaction of relatives such as José's father, at the gravesite, made her acutely regret the bones she had accidently broken since the excavation started—as their poor condition and preservation did not make their treatment easy. The underlying emotional quality of the space and the human character provided to the bones through the stories conditioned in many ways the ethics of care and precise handling of these bodies. As Samara, another volunteer, said to me during the same exhumation, "even if we treat corpses as a material thing in our everyday practice, it is inevitable that we see them as people, because that is what they are" (Samara Ibarra, Puebla, 2012). In a conversation with her one afternoon after a long morning at the mass grave, she explained to me how that day, whilst she excavated, she reflected on what she was doing and, in her words, "gained consciousness" of her actions. She looked at the corpse she had worked on for a long period of time and she imagined the person whose skeleton she excavated in the past, at the moment of his death, remarking how she envisioned what he might have been wearing. "I could see him dressed"—she affirmed—through the remnants of his clothing: through the buckles, buttons, boots and other objects, which lay with his body. Moreover, looking at his hands, she said, she could also imagine how he might have touched his family before the execution.

Intimate perceptions of the corpses were often enlivened by the ongoing touch and sight of their emerging physiognomy, as well as by the repetition of memories about the executions that some volunteers, like Samara, also had in their own families. The personal entanglement with the mass grave through the senses and the effect of learnt and owned stories propelled an active imagination of the human condition of these corpses. In such a way, the corpse transcended its qualities as a nonhuman being, which simply "swaps properties" (Latour 1999, 16) with the living—as something that is made by and, in turn, makes the human, in the sphere of scientific practice. Instead, it was conceived from the start as a human, whose remnants were always enmeshed with the image and aura of the person. This entanglement between the definition of the corpse as dead or alive was also born out of the ideological commitment of many volunteers. Such sensitivity towards the corpses shaped an even more careful scientific practice and method. The preoccupation with the excavation of the corpses also surpassed the space of the mass grave, seizing the dreams of volunteers at night. As a volunteer inside the mass grave, my own dreams were often overshadowed by an urge to overcome the difficulties I encountered in the excavation of some body parts.

For those who visited the site, the disposition and care towards the human remains on the part of the teams in Puebla and in Castuera contrasted with the extreme maltreatment registered on the corpses. In Puebla, for instance, the agitation provoked by the mass burial was recorded in a visitors' book, where people wrote messages about their impressions—something inspired by the work of the national historical memory association (ARMH) on mass graves. In the book, people often wrote comments, but also made drawings. In these representations, one could trace the "affective discharge" of the exhumation space, as Yael Navaro-Yashin (2012) has observed in relation to the remnants of conflict in northern Cyprus. In the message shown in Fig. 6.3—written by Cayetano Ibarra, the exhumation's coordinator at PREMHEx—the land, the mass grave, and the bones are portrayed as the containers of the tragedy throughout the years and of a truth only they can reveal: "the land speaks and wants to tell us sad stories about the cruel tragedy lived by these fields and holm oak trees." The gravesite, his comment suggests, listing the body parts one can see as the evidence of the crime, has its own voice as it shouts, "Here they are!" The words of the message enliven the role of the material in the construction of a history of the executions and in the articulation of a political desire—as these "residues" from violence are rendered as the "foundations of freedom" (Fig. 6.3).

Many of the comments in the book highlight how these corpses frightened and astonished people. Others retold how some neighbours who visited the site had been sick or could not eat after seeing the corpses. The violence recorded in the mass grave incited physical and intimate reactions, which unhinged people's physiology and psychology (Brennan 2004). Some recognized the political efficacy of such an affective discharge. In the light of a rapidly disintegrating economy, many feared a quick indifference towards the Civil War and postwar mass graves on the part of official institutions and society at large. One of the volunteers in Puebla, for instance, wished the sight of these bodies were never "normalized" and dispossessed of their capacity to affect people in social and political realms.

The treatment of these bodies by the perpetrators who tied them, beat them, and lined them up to be executed—as Cayetano Ibarra's drawing below imagines the execution in Puebla's visitors' book—coexisted

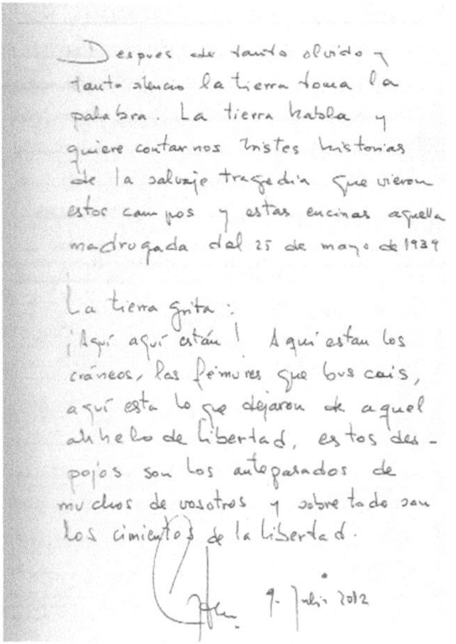

Después de tanto olvido y tanto silencio la tierra toma la palabra. La tierra habla y quiere contarnos tristes historias de la salvaje tragedia que vieron estos campos y estas encinas aquella madrugada del 25 de mayo de 1939

La tierra grita:
¡Aquí aquí están! Aquí están los cráneos, los fémures que buscáis, aquí está lo que dejaron de aquel anhelo de libertad, estos despojos son los antepasados de muchos de vosotros y sobre todo son los cimientos de la libertad.

9. Julio 2012

Translation:

After so much forgetting and silence, the land speaks. The land speaks and wants to tell us sad stories about the cruel tragedy lived by these fields and holm oak trees that early morning of 25th May 1939.

The land shouts:

"Here they are!" Here are the skulls, the femurs that you are looking for. Here you have what they left of that desire for freedom. These residues are the ancestors of many of you and above all, they are the foundations of freedom.

Fig. 6.3 Excerpt from Visitors' Book written by Cayetano Ibarra

with the gestures of precise and scrupulous management of the bones articulated by the scientific team: unearthed with screw-drivers and, later, thin sticks, when bones were visible; protected against deterioration by cautiously covering them and placing glasses filled with water inside the grave to preserve their humidity levels; carefully removed, bubble-wrapped, and classified with a number in separate carton boxes ready to be transported to the laboratory at the moment of the exhumation.

Varied methods were applied in order to protect the information contained in the bones, but most importantly to secure the skeleton's individuation and its final burial. The scientific treatment of these corpses became entrenched with the morality that surrounds death and dying in western and, more concretely, Spanish contexts. Through care, these archaeological technologies restored and dignified the corpses in the eyes of relatives, neighbours, activists and other groups who visited the exhumations.

Mortuary rites and their social importance have been widely examined in classical and contemporary texts on the anthropology of death, dying, and burial (Hertz 1960 [1909]; Metcalf and Huntington 1991; Bloch and Parry 1982; Rosaldo 1993; Seremetakis 1991; Sheper-Hughes 1992; Robben 2004). Even at the beginning of the twentieth century, studies such as Hertz's (1960, 27) were identifying how western traditions rejected a view of the body of the deceased "as carcass" and instead encouraged its "specific care [...] and correct burial; not merely for reasons of hygiene but out of a moral obligation." Quigley (1996) has described the particular processes of preparation, display, and disposal the dead body undergoes in western settings. As in other places in the Mediterranean, traditional mortuary practices in Spain have also included the appropriate washing, scenting, dressing, and laying out of the body for the wake, funeral, and its later burial in the cemetery. Nadia Seremetakis (1991, 134) has also observed how these practices bring the living closer to the soul of the dead and constitute an "extension of the kinship ethics of care and tending" when the corpse's preparation is carried out by direct relatives.

As in the southern Peloponnesus, this is also the case in Spain, where family members have looked after the dead for years, especially in rural areas. These practices have coexisted with the ongoing medicalization of death and the appearance of the morgue in the twentieth century, which placed the treatment of the corpse under expert management, reconfiguring much the of the relationship established between relatives and the dead body (ibid., see also Prior 1989). Moreover, in Spain, Catholic rituals and commemoration such as masses, prayers, and offerings have been an essential part of mourning for the deceased. Confronted with these scattered bodies, which embodied memories of violence and a lack of "funeral atonement" (Kwon 2006), families and activists perceived the work of scientists as an act that could rescue the corpses and return to them their integrity, through "laborious work" and "expertise," as people pointed out throughout the campaigns in Puebla de Alcocer and Castuera. Archaeological work, for some, secured a peaceful continuity of the deceased into their afterlives. As Luisa Cabanillas Bayón wrote in Puebla's visitors' book, to the team:

> I am really grateful to you for recovering the memory of those forgotten, who paid with their blood for their ideals. Thank you for your humane work. It will help them to rest in peace forever. With love and affection from your forever friend. (Luisa Cabanillas Bayón, Visitors' Book, Puebla de Alcocer, 2012)

Marked by the overbearing effects of the political violence registered in the mass burial and in the footprints of transgenerational despair, the exhumation was another site where the affective load of the past was felt and internalized. At the exhumation, the spectre of death was turned into a concrete reality, transforming the subjective experience of disappearance for all participants. Through its harsh materiality, the mass grave evoked a time, a place, and an event until then only vaguely imagined, and stirred other forms of knowing through *feeling*. In contact with the stories, but also the hopes and expectations of families, the site became a place through which to engage publically with the construction of history—also through the emotions. Since the executions had taken place, the absent presence of the defeated conditioned the day-to-day lives of the living and their latent war traumas. These absences also marked the agony and bitterness felt by later generations, whose need for a *postmemory* would drive them to unrelenting searches for information.

The searches will start, for many, in the archive, among its damaged documents and images, revealing a world of burdened descriptions and relations, of hurtful words and declarations. These searches will continue at the mass grave, where the material manifestation of violence on the human corpse stirred sickly sentiments and revived the pain and anxiety of the living. The archive and the mass grave surfaced as new places of transmission in which the story of those killed and their affective memory lived on in present endeavours to know the past—and then on, into the realm of the future. In the subsequent acts of reburial and commemoration, when corpses entered the cemetery, a third space emerged for the transcendence of these stories of repression. Here, other familial, personal, and political desires loomed in relation to the identification and memorialisation of the war killed and disappeared.

Notes

1. At a later exhumation, in the village of Fregenal de la Sierra in September 2012, Fernando Brazo, one of the men whose father had been buried in the mass grave in the cemetery of the village, poignantly said to us in an interview: "Those who were killed at least died, but the ones who stayed [mainly referring to his mother] remained dead whilst still alive" (Fernando Brazo, Fregenal de la Sierra, 2012).

2. *La matanza* is popular event in Extremadura where a year-old pig is sacrificed to produce meat for its owners. It is common for those who kill and butcher the animal to get together before the killing in order to eat a hearty breakfast accompanied by alcoholic drinks such as moonshine or liquor to warm up in the cold winter months.

References

Agustí i Roca, Carme, and Concepción Mir. 2005. Delincuencia patrimonial y justicia penal durante el Franquismo (1939-1951): una incursión en la marginación. In *Pobreza, marginación, delincuencia y políticas sociales bajo el franquismo*, ed. Josep Gelonch Solé, Concepción Mir, and Carme Agustí i Roca. Lleida: Universitat de Lleida. Servicio de Publicaciones.

Agustí i Roca, Carme, Josep Gelonch Solé, and Concepción Mir. 2005. *Pobreza, marginación, delincuencia y políticas sociales bajo el franquismo*. Lleida: Universitat de Lleida. Servicio de Publicaciones.

Bloch, Maurice, and Jonathan Parry. 1982. *Death and the Regeneration of Life*. Cambridge: Cambridge University Press.

Brennan, Teresa. 2004. *The Transmission of Affect*. Ithaca: Cornell University Press.

Burton, Antoinette M. 2003. *Dwelling in the Archive: Women Writing House, Home, and History in Late Colonial India*. New York: Oxford University Press.

Caruth, Cathy. 1995. *Trauma: Explorations in Memory*. Baltimore: Johns Hopkins University Press.

Caruth, Cathy. 1996. *Unclaimed Experience: Trauma, Narrative, and History*. Baltimore: Johns Hopkins University Press.

Chaves Palacios, Julián. 2005. Franquismo: prisiones y prisioneros. *Pasado y Memoria. Revista de Historia Contemporánea* 4: 27–47.

Cho, Grace M. 2008. *Haunting the Korean Diaspora: Shame, Secrecy and the Forgotten War*. Minneapolis: University of Minnesota Press.

Cobo Romero, Francisco. 2005. *Represión y persecución de minorías y disidentes en las dictaduras fascistas europeas del período de entreguerras: los apoyos sociales y la colaboración de ciudadanos comunes. La Alemania Nazi y la España franquista*, ed. Josep Gelonch Solé, Concepción Mir, and Carme Agustí i Roca. Lleida: Universitat de Lleida. Servicio de Publicaciones.

Das, Veena. 1996. Language and the Body: Transactions in the Construction of Pain. *Daedalus, Social Suffering* 125 (1): 65–91.

Das, Veena. 2007. *Life and Words: Violence and the Descent into the Ordinary*. Berkeley: University of California Press.

Derrida, Jacques. 1996. *Archive Fever: A Freudian Impression*. Chicago and London: University of Chicago Press.

Domanska, Ewa. 2005. Toward the Archaeontology of the Dead Body. *Rethinking History* 9 (4): 389–413.
Gordon, Avery. 1997. *Ghostly Matters: Haunting and the Sociological Imagination*. Minneapolis: University of Minnesota Press.
Hertz, Robert, Claudia Needham, and Rodney Needham. 1960. *Death and the Right Hand*, trans. Rodney and Claudia Needham. London: Cohen & West.
Hirsch, Marianne. 2012. *The Generation of Postmemory: Writing and Visual Culture After the Holocaust*. New York, NY and Chichester: Columbia University Press.
Kwon, Heonik. 2006. *After the Massacre: Commemoration and Consolation in Ha My and My Lai*. Berkeley, CA and London: University of California Press.
Latour, Bruno. 1999. *Pandora's Hope: Essays on the Reality of Science Studies*. Cambridge, MA and London: Harvard University Press.
Metcalf, Peter, and Richard Huntington. 1991. *Celebrations of Death: The Anthropology of Mortuary Ritual*. Cambridge: Cambridge University Press.
Miñarro, Anna, and Teresa Morandi. 2013. *Trauma y transmisión: Efectos de la guerra del 36, la posguerra, la dictadura y la transición en la subjetividad de los ciudadanos*. Barcelona: Xoroi Edicions.
Montero García, Feliciano. 2005. Asistencia social, catolicismo y franquismo: la actuación de acción católica en la posguerra. In *Pobreza, marginación, delincuencia y políticas sociales bajo el franquismo*, ed. Josep Gelonch Solé, Concepción Mir, and Carme Agustí i Roca. Lleida: Universitat de Lleida.
Muñoz, Giménez, and Maria del Carmen. 2009. La Asistencia Social en Sevilla: del Auxilio de Invierno al Auxilio Social (1936–1939), *Hispania Nova. Revista de Historia Contemporánea, 9*.
Navaro-Yashin, Yael. 2012. *The Make-Believe Space: Affective Geography in a Postwar Polity*. Durham, NC: Duke University Press.
Portelli, Alessandro. 2003. *The Order Has Been Carried Out: History, Memory, and Meaning of a Nazi Massacre in Rome*. New York: Palgrave Macmillan.
Quigley, Christine. 1996. *The Corpse: A History*. Jefferson, London: McFarland.
Renshaw, Layla. 2011. *Exhuming Loss: Memory, Materiality and Mass Graves of the Spanish Civil War*. Walnut Creek: Left Coast.
Robben, Antonius C.G.M. 2004. *Death, Mourning, and Burial: A Cross-Cultural Reader*. Oxford: Blackwell.
Rosaldo, Renato. 1993. *Culture & Truth: The Remaking of Social Analysis*. London: Routledge.
Sanford, Victoria. 2003. *Buried Secrets: Truth and Human Rights in Guatemala*. New York, NY: Palgrave Macmillan.
Scheper-Hughes, Nancy. 1992. *Death Without Weeping: The Violence of Everyday Life in Brazil*. Berkeley: University of California Press.
Seremetakis, Nadia C. 1991. *The Last Word: Women, Death, and Divination in Inner Mani*. Chicago: University of Chicago Press.

Steedman, Carolyn. 2001. *Dust*. Manchester: Manchester University Press.
Steedman, Carolyn. 2008. Romance in the Archive. The Ontology of the Archive Symposium, ESRC Centre for Research on Socio-Cultural Change, Manchester.
Ysás Solanes, Pere, and Carme Molinero Ruiz. 2003. Las condiciones de vida y laborales durante el primer franquismo. La subsistencia ¿un problema político. *Ayer* 52: 255–282.

CHAPTER 7

Reburial and Commemoration

Since the beginning of the exhumation movement in 2000, parallel acts of commemoration have occurred as part of a collective effort to address and memorialise the war and postwar past, all over Spain. Acts such as the one that has been celebrated in Castuera every year since 2006—discussed in Chap. 4—emerged as communal spaces, on the margins of state action, where distinct generations met to remember disappeared and executed relatives and to publicly denounce a history of violence and pain. Commemoration has become a decentralized practice (Kwon 2006), promoted and fulfilled by civil society groups—members of second, third, and fourth generations. These acts vigorously demand further involvement from local and national authorities in the search and recovery of the corpses of the defeated and their remembrance. This lack of a state commitment around the atonement of Francoist crimes also shaped the experience of returning and reburying the human remains found in the mass graves of Castuera and Puebla de Alcocer, as well as their commemoration.

Unlike in other contexts, such as Bosnia (Wagner 2008) or Argentina, where the search for and identification of human remains from the conflict was endorsed by state actors or, in the case of the Balkans, by the international community, in Spain, those who search for their blood and "political" kin are liable for the scientific analysis of human remains and their reburial. Though the projects in Castuera and Puebla de Alcocer received financial aid from the Ministry of the Presidency, which in many cases covered DNA typing, the central government provided neither

Z. Aragüete-Toribio, *Producing History in Spanish Civil War Exhumations*, World Histories of Crime, Culture and Violence,
DOI 10.1007/978-3-319-61270-6_7

logistic aid nor general support for the project. The funerary rituals and idioms that emerged in connection to their reburial were filled with expressions of grief and rights claims over their historical recognition. In the two cases discussed throughout the book, as well as others documented in Extremadura, identification and reburial were further affected by the condition in which many of these corpses were found inside the mass graves. Their corroded physiognomy greatly impacted on the way in which the individuation of corpses was carried out and influenced the choice of burial performed in different locations. This last chapter examines the act of returning the corpses exhumed to the ground of the cemetery, focusing on the experience of three reburial projects. In so doing, it explores the distinct moralities at play in these endeavours, tracing the meanings and material outcomes these reburials acquire in connection to the motivations and desires of families, activists, and the state.

Identification and Collective Reburial

As in other post-conflict scenarios, the act of reburying the bodies found in war and postwar mass graves in Spain is preceded by the individuation of each corpse, the anthropological study of the bones—of their antemortem, perimortem, and postmortem traits—and later, DNA testing and matching. Sarah Wagner (2008, 2014) has discussed how DNA identification reattaches a name to a set of human remains and associates it again with the family to whom the person executed was connected. The search for, identification, and return of corpses to families has united scientific practice and social expectations in the restoration of disrupted kinship relations. It has also further entangled the lives of survivors with the aspirations of the state. In particular instances, such as the Srebrenica genocide, authors like Wagner have pointed out how DNA testing has become a key technology that "speaks to the state's capacities to regulate and respond to the need of its citizens" (2008, 255). In her analysis, however, Wagner is critical about how such use of DNA identification and individuation techniques reasserts states' authority in a landscape of different political claims and conceals previous forms of governmental inaction or disdain in situations of emergency—like in the event of war or a natural disaster (ibid.). This "technology of repair", as Wagner calls it, is placed at the mercy of political agendas (ibid.). In these contexts, the use of an advanced identification technology such as DNA turns sovereign power into an authority that allegedly *cares* whilst concealing past negligence, especially in the aftermath of extreme violence—political, ethnic, religious, or otherwise. In Spain, the lack of a state commitment to exhuming and identifying those killed by Francoist groups—first during the Socialist Party mandate (2004–2011) and after 2011, with the Popular Party—has placed the individuation of corpses and their DNA analysis in the hands of independent scientific teams and associations since the turn of the twenty-first century.

DNA testing has played an important role in the identification of human remains found in Spanish mass graves, especially in cases where conditions were most favourable—i.e., where bodies are well preserved and living relatives can still be found today after so many years. Due to the temporal divide between the killings and the exhumation, forensic scientists working on war and postwar mass graves in Spain have advised that DNA testing cannot be taken in isolation and instead needs to be "targeted" or related to other types of presumptive and osteological identification attained through the cross-referencing of archival sources, testimonies, and the osteological study of bones and dentures (Rios et al. 2010). Some case studies such as Rios et al. (2010, e27) have further highlighted that identification processes in Spain depend on numerous factors, just as in other international contexts, which determine their successful accomplishment. Elements such as the number of bodies found in the mass grave, their preservation and related belongings, the methods available for their analysis, and the "quantity and quality" of antemortem data; or "the availability of financial support and living relatives" for DNA analysis are key to securing a positive identification.

A close look at the reports produced from excavations carried out in distinct geographical locations of the Spanish territory by different scientific teams reveals the idiosyncratic character of such identification processes, which are determined by the variations of each burial and social context. In some cases, when positive identification can be achieved, DNA results can confirm existing hypotheses drawn from presumptive data about the identity of individuals found, for instance, in archives, especially when dealing with large groups (see Rios et al. 2010 for an example). In others, it can act as the only method for matching the identity of the victim to that of his or her relatives, particularly when there is a small number of corpses—see for instance the case of the exhumation in Aibar-Oibar (Navarra) discussed by Etxeberría et al. (2012), where the absence of antemortem data led to DNA testing to find a match between the four bodies encountered and the families present at the excavation.

In further cases, in which DNA proof cannot be obtained—due the poor conservation of bones, an absence of living relatives of the deceased or a lack of funds—only forms of osteological and presumptive identification can be performed.

As Berta Silva—a member of the excavation team from the Universidad Autónoma de Madrid that was led by biologist Luis Rios and who has also collaborated with the Sociedad de Ciencias Aranzadi and with Laura Muñoz Encinar in numerous exhumations in Extremadura—explained to me, the cases they have dealt with in exhumations principally in northern Spain, have allowed her team to complete a DNA analysis of human remains regularly. In fact, as she observes, individual identification through DNA is performed every time it is possible and not only when families demand it, as it is "part of their working procedure" (personal communication with Berta Silva). The possibility of obtaining a positive identification of the dead, in particular through the certainty provided by DNA testing, has prompted a re-encounter between numerous families and their kin more than seventy years after their deaths. As Berta further described, many families claimed their relatives' human remains in order to inter them in private familial gravesites. Nonetheless, the archaeologist clarified that in the cases she had worked on, a common mausoleum was usually built to accommodate identified, partially identified, and unknown human remains. There, corpses, especially those whose families cannot be located, would be buried in individual coffins, with relevant scientific information about their human traits, ready for future exhumation and identification.

For instance, in cases such as the excavation of the Central Prison of Valdenoceda in Burgos carried out by scientists from Aranzadi, the Universidad Autónoma de Madrid and with the support of ARMH, where a vast number of corpses were exhumed and analysed, the families' association took responsibility for the burial and commemoration of those that could not be returned to their families. Many of these corpses were identified through existing presumptive and osteological data, but a positive identification could not be concluded, as many relatives were not found. Nonetheless, volunteers from the association continue, still today, searching for relatives in order to secure the DNA analysis of corpses—as the blog dedicated to the exhumation describes (http://exhumacionvaldenoceda.com). Time has dispersed families and made these searches arduous in the present. In other instances, it has also eroded bones and objects and damaged telling documents that can shed light on the identity of those captured and their killings—as in the case of the prisoners of Castuera concentration camp. Such contingencies are contemplated in the exhumations' protocol issued in September 2011 by the outgoing PSOE, which further connects questions about the identification of the Civil War and postwar executed to their final fate and resting place. As part E of the last section of the protocol advises:

E) Final Resting Place of Human Remains

Once human remains are studied and identified, depending on whether they have been identified or not, their burial will proceed as follows:

1. Identified [human remains]: families will receive them and perform the ceremony they consider appropriate.
2. Not identified: [human remains] will be inhumed at the cemetery of the location where the mass grave is located. The most adequate containers will be used, according to the recommendations of conservation and restoration experts. Each body will be buried individually, together with their personal belongings, with an identification that allows their location in future exhumations. This identification should include in all cases their case-study number.

> Likewise, authorisation from the Autonomous Community or relevant Local Entity will be required for the transportation of human remains as well as for their re-inhumation or cremation. (Excerpt from the Exhumation Practice Protocol, Spanish Ministry of the Presidency, *Boletín Oficial del Estado*, 2011: 101, 917)

Hence, the re-inhumation of corpses from Civil War and postwar mass graves in Spain is largely influenced by the precepts of their identification as well as the legal context of the place where they are interred.[1] Authors such as Wagner (2014) have observed that the complexities encountered in some processes of identification—for instance in reference to her study of commingled remains in Bosnian secondary mass graves—have in fact generated the creation of innovative burial practices and forms to cater to the dead and its mourning socially. This was often the case in Extremadura. Certainly some exhumations, as in the case of that in the village of Villasbuenas de Gata (Cáceres) (personal communication with Laura Muñoz), have resulted in successful DNA matches and identification. Nonetheless, in the exhumations in which I participated in Castuera and Puebla de Alcocer, several factors hampered DNA analysis and anthropological examination. In Castuera, uncertainty over the identities of the bodies found, and an absence of clues about the killings in the civil registry and of direct relatives rendered identification unlikely. In Puebla de Alcocer, it was the state of many of the corpses reduced to osseous splinters and also the difficulty in locating all families that led to the same problem.

From the beginning, the reburial of the corpses found in Puebla and Castuera had been conceived as a collective act, since a positive identification seemed so far-fetched. In Puebla, where there were some families connected to the men in the mass graves, identification was perceived as a time-consuming and costly procedure. Having only located half of the number of families of the 40 men he identified on the files of the official registry—some of whom did not want to be involved in the exhumation—DNA typing would require more time to search for other families and funds. Moreover, José acknowledged that in the event of a DNA test, he would almost certainly obtain the corpses of his grandfather and his granduncle, but wondered what would happen to the remaining unidentified corpses, which belonged to other neighbours from Puebla. There was a sense of urgency with regard to fulfilling a much-desired end: to bury these human remains at the village cemetery, as many relatives from older generations were quickly passing away.

For José, a collective burial in a mausoleum, like the one in Fig. 7.1, was a fair option, since all of the bodies could rest and be commemorated as a group. For many of those to whom I spoke, burying and mourning all the corpses together made sense, since, in José's words, "they died together, [had] been together and [would] remain together in the cemetery, where they should be" (José Sánchez-Paniagua, Puebla 2012). For other relatives like Pablo Trenado Cabanillas, a collective burial meant that all could be gathered in the same place, especially considering the manner in which some corpses had "turned out"—fractured and worn away (Pablo Trenado Cabanillas, Puebla 2012). Their collective reburial involved the design of a hollow structure where they would be stored in individual coffins with a case number, but without a name attached to them. As the protocol suggests, they would be prepared for examination should any relative wish to identify the bones of their dead kin in the future. Their unnamed boxes inside the crypt would symbolize the identity of the many men who were killed in Puebla's trenches. The names found on the death certificates from the archive and corroborated by testimonies would be carved on the stone that covered the exterior of the monolith (see Fig. 7.1). An excerpt from a conversation with José, his

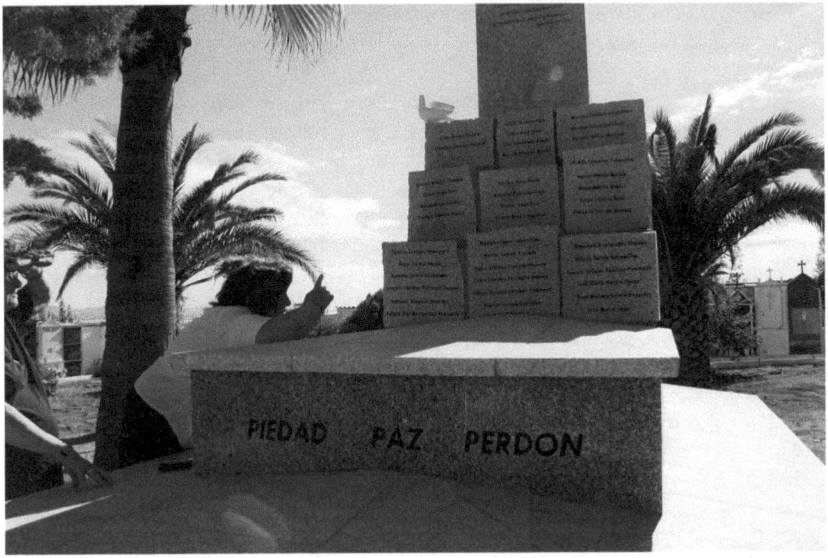

Fig. 7.1 Mausoleum in the cemetery of Puebla de Alcocer where the 42 bodies exhumed rest. The names of those killed at the mass grave are listed on the top and the inscription at bottom reads: "*Compassion, Peace, Forgiveness*"

sister Consuelo, and Esperanza Muga Blasco during a visit to Esperanza's house in the summer of 2012, elucidates how the idea of these communal internments was negotiated—and what happened when they came into contact with individual wishes for a positive identification—when people imagined how the human remains of their ancestors would be retuned after the exhumation:

ZA: Esperanza, what does it mean to you to recover the remains of your relatives?

EM: Well, what I don't know is… how do they know which bones belong to one family and which to another? The bones, I mean, it must be because of the bones …

ZA: Yes, after they have been exhumed, it is the archaeologist who studies them and tests them.

EM: But bones, I don't know what evidence must be in bones…

CSP: Did my brother not mention to you how it will be done? Did you not tell her, José?

JSP: Yes, yes I told her but she might not remember now … We will build a common burial site in the cemetery. The bones will come out from the ground where they are. They will take them to Cáceres, where they will be analysed. They will classify them and place them inside small numbered boxes and bring them back to the cemetery. At the cemetery, we will build a mausoleum where they will all be buried together. So you will not receive the human remains of your father, grandfather, or uncles. They are all going to be together in the mausoleum. You will know your family is there, but for now, you will not know exactly who they are.

EM: [to José and Consuelo] And your grandfather, will he be there too?

JSP: Yes, our grandfather too.

CSP: Your father's bones will be all together because they will know which bones belong to each body. But you will not know which body is your father's because in order to know that you need a DNA test and this costs a great deal of money.

JSP: And time …

CSP: Let's imagine you say tomorrow "I want to know and I am going to pay to identify my father". Then they will take them out, because each one is classified in a box, and they will find out.
(Esperanza Muga Blasco; José Sánchez-Paniagua and Consuelo Sánchez-Paniagua, Puebla, 2012)

The difficulties faced in the process of identification altered the expectations of some families, such as Esperanza's, who, on several occasions before and during the exhumation, made clear her hope of fully identifying her three relatives—father, uncle, and grandfather—at the mass grave. Throughout the campaign, Esperanza was eager to learn what tests archaeologists would run on the bodies to reveal her relatives' identity. She had asked about the possibility of a DNA analysis on several occasions after my first visit to her house with José and Consuelo. Even when we spoke about it during our visit, she seemed familiar with the term, demonstrating the wide reach of this scientific method and its presumed efficacy in many social milieus. This was not the first time someone had manifested a clear familiarity with DNA technology.

Many had referred to it at different exhumations, associating the sight of the human remains with their forensic meanings and treatment. Many members of the scientific team attributed this local knowledge of practices such as DNA testing to their regular presence in mass media (e.g., in series such as *CSI* or the news). Their observations coincide with the view of some authors like Jacque Lynn Foltyn (2008), who have pointed out the role of the corpse and its forensic treatment at the centre of popular culture productions. The ascent of the dead body and its scientific meanings as a theme of public interest, Foltyn argues, has also reasserted the authority of DNA evidence and examination.

Explaining the limitations of these identification methods, especially in difficult contexts such as that of Puebla's mass grave, contested the image of outmost certitude that some cultural representations of such scientific activity generated. In our last weekend in Puebla, I accompanied Laura Muñoz to Esperanza's house one more time. It was clear by then that a DNA test was not really an option. Laura explained to her that an individual identification had to be considered a "remote possibility", since acquiring additional information that could help to individuate those in groups that were in better conditions—in order to perform a DNA analysis—was extremely complex. Moreover, Laura explained that many of the bones needed for a positive DNA extraction, like dentures or femurs, were missing. The archaeologist added, though, that if indicators that associated a corpse with a specific family emerged during her study of the human remains—for instance, they knew Esperanza's father had a limp—then a DNA test might be carried out on that concrete set of human remains. Esperanza aspired to recuperate her relatives' human remains but also recognized the difficulties that the dearth of information and the uncertainty over these men's antemortem traits and their executions—as the archaeologist explained—had caused in the identification process.

Collective reburials of individuated human remains are ensnared with the predicaments of time, place, and conservation and the social politics around these war and postwar dead in Extremadura. These internments prompted the creation of new spaces of remembrance, in which a distinct commemorative culture emerged. The act of re-inhuming these human remains together celebrated the individual identities of the defeated but also their common histories, stimulating the imagination of a new community—in Benedict Anderson's terms (1999)—of mourners around the human remains. In a different article about the identification of MIA soldiers in the USA, anthropologist Sarah Wagner (2013) has discussed how DNA technology has contributed to identifying the bodies buried in the Vietnam crypt of the Tomb of the Unknowns in Arlington's cemetery, redefining the modes and meanings of national commemoration in the country. Collective burials, such as the one performed in Puebla de Alcocer and also in places such as Castuera and others, recognized the individual identity of each of the men found in the mass graves, but also turned the corpses into symbols for the making of a collective history and identity. Families, activists, and sometimes local political representatives came together in the organization and realization of these events, manifesting the heterogeneity of intentions and desires at play in the creation of these funerary vestiges and acts of reburial.

Reburial in the Cemetery

Throughout fieldwork, most families and activists I met in Extremadura understood the reburial of the human remains in the village or town cemetery as a way of honouring the defeated. They often recalled left-wing followers in mass graves for the loathsome way in which they were buried, emphasizing their displaced condition. These men and women were still today lying on roadsides and outside of cemeteries "just like dogs" (*tirados como perros*). José Sánchez-Paniagua, for instance, said to me on various occasions that people should be interred inside the cemetery, as only "animals" where buried outside. Likewise, indifference towards these deaths or a refusal to recover a relative's human remains from the mass graves on the part of some families, for instance, in Puebla, was strongly criticized by some, as an attitude that demonstrated a lack of integrity and care for the family ancestor. Returning these dead to the cemetery constituted a dislocated act in time to restore their legitimacy and humanity, but it also complied with a certain "morality of death"—to evoke Heonik Kwon's (2006) expression—based on the belief that these bodies, as kin, fellow militant or neighbour, had endured a form of "*undignified*" death and burial for years.

As in the case of the familial rituals and commemoration around those killed and buried in mass graves in Vietnam, which Kwon (2006, 2008) discusses, these internments, their design and commemorative rituals aimed to re-signify the negative meanings associated with their violent deaths. Situating these dead bodies inside the realm of the cemetery bestowed upon the human remains a sacred and solemn character. As an established place for the dead in each locality, the cemetery was not only conceived as a space where "good deaths" found their burial but also a place that secured a respected afterlife for the dead, from the point of view of the community of the living. Municipal cemeteries have been imbued with different secular and religious connotations from their origins in the eighteenth and nineteenth centuries—when they were built after burial conditions under churches' grounds became insalubrious (Granjel and Carreras Pachón 2004). In Extremadura, as elsewhere, they also acquired dynamic meanings in connection to the social relations that determined their changing landscapes—as some authors have observed of similar funerary compounds (Rugg 2003; Buckham 2003). In past years, the transformation of these sites has been apparent as multiple memorials and monuments have been erected to commemorate the Republican dead.

Historian Susan Buckham (2003) has emphasized the important role of cemetery constructions such as memorials in the representation of the dead and in the portrayal of the social affiliations and familial identities of the bereaved. Within the cemetery, memorials have allowed the bereaved to express and feel their unique connection to the deceased in particular social contexts. The need for recognition and reburial of the war defeated is entangled with what many relatives and activists see as a right to have a commemorative space inside the cemetery's boundaries. That Puebla's town mayor considered the mass burials in the trenches, in his words, an "anomaly", was prompted by the same belief and wish to gather these uprooted bodies in the cemetery, to create a space where their deaths could be grieved as part of the village community. For some, even their return to the cemetery was controversial, making their reburial a matter of dispute between families and local political authorities. For instance, relatives like Ángel Sayabera in Castuera had always wished for the construction of a monolith in remembrance of those who, like his mother, father, and brothers, had disappeared during and after the occupation of the village. In an interview, Ángel told me that he knew finding and identifying his relatives' remains through DNA analysis would be highly unlikely, because they could be anywhere among the vast number of prisoners buried at the back of Castuera cemetery or in mines next to the Camp. In addition, at the cemetery, many corpses had been removed in construction and renovation works throughout the years, making their location even more troublesome. Ángel believed that since he, like many other families from the village, might never find his relatives' human remains, a monolith should be built in or outside the cemetery where their kin could mourn. Ángel had wanted a monument even before the exhumation had taken place. When he and others wrote to the socialist town mayor in Castuera before the 2011 election to suggest the building of a monolith, the town mayor expressed his unease with the instalment of the structure in the cemetery, arguing that "the Republic had nothing to do with cemetery" (Ángel Sayabera, Llera 2011). Ángel explained the town mayor argued that putting a plaque on the wall of the village's town hall would be a more appropriate form of commemoration. For Ángel this suggestion betrayed a lack of consideration of grieving families' needs. As he described:

> I wrote to the town mayor and told him that perhaps the Republic and the cemetery may have nothing to do with one another, but our dead and the cemetery have everything to do with each other, you know? They wanted us to put a small plaque on the town hall's door. I said: 'what would you think if all of us, pariahs (*apestados*), took crowns and bundles of flowers to the town hall?' It seems commonsensical that this should be done in the cemetery. (Ángel Sayabera, Llera 2011)

The political meanings attached to the human remains of the defeated, their connection to a pre-war past, and the Republican political aspirations of younger generations in the present triggered an anxiety around the memorialisation of these dead and their history, especially on the part of many in governing circles. These attitudes towards the commemoration of the defeated, for some like Ángel, perpetuated the treatment of these families as outcasts—a feeling experienced by many relatives that, since the postwar period, had endured the stigma of other members of the community. These anxieties were also felt when, in the process of reburial, collective decisions were made about the location, design, and composition of memorials built to re-inter exhumed human remains in the cemetery. In many cases, as Ángel's example above also denotes, the visibility of the tombstones became a central issue in negotiations between families, activists, and political representatives about the configuration, exhibition, and reception of the monument. After all, these monoliths and the bones contained inside their vaults indexed a traumatic part of each locality's history, inscribing memories of violence, absence, and loss on the landscape of the cemetery. Having a permanent place that pointed to this part of the village's past, especially inside the burial ground, awakened the angst and disquiet of some, who still feared remembrance of the conflict and, in particular, the stories of those who suffered defeat.

In places such as Puebla de Alcocer, where the village's town hall backed the exhumation and reburial project, the space designated for the mausoleum was one of the most central areas of the cemetery. Many, including the village's socialist leader, envisaged the reburial as an act of justice and equality. As he explained to me, it was "wrong" that a community should have some of their neighbours buried in the middle of the countryside in the twenty-first century (Manuel Moreno Delgado, Puebla 2012). For the town mayor, returning these bodies to the village's cemetery complied with a morality and obligation intimately connected to a notion of modernity and progress. Marking the space of the cemetery with this construction materialised a political wish to pay tribute to these deaths, but also symbolized the triumph of democracy.

In such a way, throughout the process of creating the monument, designed by PREMHEx exhumations' coordinator, Cayetano Ibarra, Cayetano and the town mayor envisaged the mausoleum in a focal zone of the compound—a not too crowded area, surrounded by palm trees that accentuated the majestic look of the memorial (see Fig. 7.1). Its design and salient placement also conformed to a need, as José Sánchez-Panigua and the town mayor agreed, to "make history" in Puebla de Alcocer—José, for instance, believed that the place were the mass grave was located, in the countryside, should also be marked as part of the same effort to register past events on the village landscape. Recalling Paul Connerton's (1989) practices of remembrance, these reburial designs act as "inscribing practices" that seek to evoke and incorporate the story and identity of the defeated and their families in the collective imagination of the village. In Puebla, the granite structure was presided over by an epitaph that conjured the personal struggle experienced throughout generations and a message that spoke of a desire for reconciliation. On top of the mausoleum one can read: "We opened your mass graves and closed our wounds. We write your names and recover your memory". At the bottom, a succinct caption summons readers to: "Compassion, Peace, Forgiveness".

As a structure designed to empower familial mourning, the memorial in Puebla de Alcocer shared many features with the tombstones of other deceased from the community. Like on the other gravestones (and in a similar manner to the Vietnam Memorial Wall of names), listing the names of those killed was an essential part of recalling who they were, especially considering their identities had been misrepresented in so many state files. As Thomas Laqueur (1994) has observed in relation to the commemoration of soldiers who died during the First War World, the hypernormalism or recurrent use of names on the inscriptions of the individual internments and collective memorials to the fallen aimed to represent the "collectivity of the dead" and to provide a primary site of mourning for families who could not recover the human remains of their kin. The monolith in Puebla fixed the names of the executed to a concrete place, making their identities visible again whilst creating novel affiliations among living neighbours. The co-existence of these names on the surface of the stone pointed to each individual story of depravation of dead and living relatives. It also, however, brought different families together—who might not otherwise meet—in a pressing collective endeavour for reparation. The lengthy register of names and the eulogies etched on the stone spoke of a communal and familial desire for historical and social acknowledgement that challenged the socio-political status quo around the Francoist past ("we write your name and we recover your memory"). Inspired by other reburial projects in Extremadura, such as that realized in the village of Llerena, the monument in Puebla spoke to the past struggle of these men and the present struggle between living relatives and the national administration.

In other cases, some of these memorial designs stood out for their originality and the significance they acquired as new technologies of historical enunciation. For instance, in the case of the reburial monument envisioned by some of those who promoted the exhumation in Castuera, the idea for the memorial was inspired by the techno-scientific finds of the excavation. In Castuera, AMECADEC commissioned a young architect, José Milara, who had also collaborated as a volunteer throughout the exhumation campaign, to design the memorial structure. Though the design has not yet been agreed and the memorial has not been built, the initial concept—characterized by its high-tech design (Fig. 7.2)—aimed to remain intricately enmeshed with the scientific, political, and familial experiences of the mass grave and its memorialisation. Following AMECADEC's brief, Milara set out to create a design inspired by the association's wish to bury each corpse individually, and, just as in other cases, with their relevant anthropological information, to enable future DNA identification. In so doing, the project, as in other artistic ventures

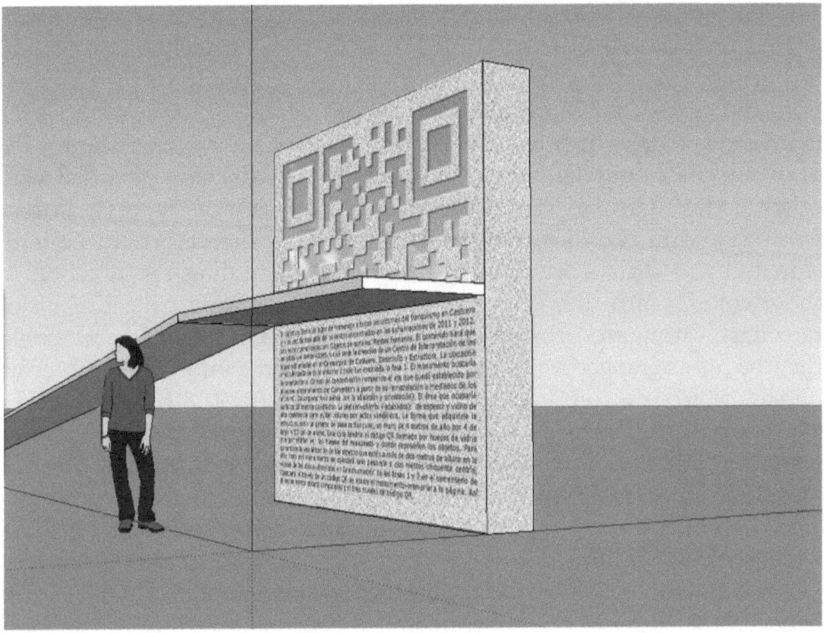

Fig. 7.2 Initial idea for a mausoleum in Castuera cemetery to bury the bodies exhumed in 2011 and 2012. The association chose a different design in the end, which was inaugurated in April 2017. Courtesy of José Milara

elsewhere, such as the case of the "etoy" project in Zürich discussed by Maja Petrović-Šteger (2012), rendered the human remains of the defeated as a site of information storage (ibid.). Here dead bodies and their belongings were objects of mourning and remembrance but also cognitive props or fragments for an exploration into the village's history of repression.

For Milara, the association's guidelines evoked an idea away from the classical monolith and more closely connected to the multidimensional features of a QR code, where "pixels, squares, and pieces such as those in a puzzle eventually form a whole image" (José Milara, Castuera 2012). The memorial would have two façades. A large cement QR code would compose the first side, with compartments made out of glass to include human remains and objects. The second side would have a footbridge to allow people to access the top sections of the four-metre memorial.

The bottom area would include a list of names of all those who disappeared in Castuera. José's design aimed to move from the concrete to the generic and vice versa. In the project, the meaning of the exhumation and history of repression as a whole would be represented by a matrix QR code, which was complemented with information about each body and its belongings in its "drawers" or "pixels" and provided with other codes. Through the QR codes, archaeological reports, history writings and images of the process, corpses and objects would be individuated and their story broadly disseminated, turning the function of the memorial into that of an archive of particular and collective histories. Each QR figure—the complete image as well as smaller ones—could then be photographed with a mobile device and the information accessed on-site or from a website. As Petrović-Šteger (2012, 80) has observed about the "etoy" project, this way of representing the dead is paradigmatic of "a moment in which the dead are routinely managed through reassociation, classification and identification technologies" worldwide. The monument would hence have a physical presence in the cemetery and also a digital form on the internet—encouraging a type of displaced memorialisation. This novel technology of remembrance would exist between the realm of the concrete and the virtual, distributing, as some have noted, "the 'life-force' of the dead person" (Petrović-Šteger 2012, 78; Gell 1999) into other realms and future generations.

This historical approach to the memorial also influenced the physical location of the monument. In his study of the social life of Holocaust memorial sites over time, James Young (1993, 7) has observed how such monuments have impacted on spaces, becoming a "point of reference" "which create[s] meaning in land and recollection," especially at the moment of their creation. In Milara's design, the space of the monolith occupies that of Mass Grave 1 in the cemetery. For the architect, situating the memorial in the same place as the mass grave defines the history of the mass burial in correlation with other war vestiges like the concentration Camp, challenging the spatial disposition of the cemetery. The position and orientation of the monolith, whose location faces that of the Camp on a straight diagonal, attempts to encumber the cemetery's apparent order and signify the latent ruination of the war past in the locality. Its material semblance was created to transform the landscape of the cemetery, among the other familial mausoleums and tombstones in the burial ground. Moreover, the monument, as a funerary construction, aimed to connect with the stories and personal needs of family members such as Ángel Sayabera and others. Features such as the engraved names under the footbridge intended to reinforce the personal and familial value of the object whilst accentuating its proximity. The monument, as Milara expressed, would conform to families' desires, providing a site that is at once a repository of past stories and a concrete place where the dead and missing can be mourned. As he explained:

> When thinking about the location, the most appropriate place I thought of was that where most remains were found. I then thought of playing with the orthogonal order found in the cemetery … You enter the cemetery and think that everything has always been ok and tidy; that there were always good relations and no one ever did anything bad, but it is not like this. [The place] inspired me to change this orthogonality, so that the object, being so closed to the concentration Camp, broke with the linearity of the cemetery and hence, of the dictatorship and transitional years; to begin to highlight landmarks that had not been considered in the village until recently, such as the concentration Camp. The monument at once remembers all the families that did not have a place to go and cry for the deaths [of their relatives], whilst it also connects the viewer with the Camp and even other sites […]. Although we incorporate innovative elements such as the QR codes, we must understand that many people feel closer to what is tangible. So for instance, the simple fact of having the names engraved on the granite stone makes [the monument] feel closer, like you even want to touch it. (José Milara, Castuera 2012)

The technical design proposed by Milara was, nonetheless, still problematic for some—even for the architect—who feared families might not be able to identify with such an intricate construction. The design of the memorial was enmeshed at all times in a process of negotiation in which the expectations of distinct groups and generations conferred and collided. Memorial designs are ultimately fraught with the manifold desires of local groups administering the construction process and, above all, with families' petitions. For instance, when the architect presented the design to members of AMECADEC, there were divisions about the aesthetic value of the monument and its functionality. According to Milara, some people agreed that the object should be built, because it was a "work of art". The majority argued that, before a decision was made, families should be consulted on whether they felt comfortable with the memorial's design. For the architect, the most important question was to think about the construction in collaboration with those who would use it most, placing an emphasis on the "wants and feelings of the relatives who [had] waited for so many years" for a place to grieve. The object of commemoration, according to Milara, should be a response to these families' demands, instead of solely to the requests of groups or local administrations that might contribute to the realization of the commemorative project. As Milara added in our interview: "for all we know, families might just want a commemorative plaque or no monument at all" (José Milara, Castuera 2012).

This exploration into memorial building expounded the central role familial needs and action play in peripheral forms of commemoration outside of state response. Such processes also evidenced the divergent positions and the sense of entitlement that influenced decision-making around the commemoration of the history of the war and the deaths of left-wing Republicans. As Young (1993) has also pointed out, memorials can elucidate how the interactions of different opinions confer and collide to settle upon what the memorial should communicate and who should really dictate that message. Ideological, economic, and personal interests tainted the tone of many of these debates, unravelling the messiness of the "'us' who remembers and commemorates" (Jelin and Langland 2003, 15) in these decentralized settings. Following the process of construction of these monuments evidenced the type of relations that produced them. During fieldwork, other memorial projects exemplified how commemoration can increase familial distress and strain the relationship between the members of historical memory groups, as well as between these groups and the local and national administrations.

In 2011, I followed the construction of another memorial in the village of Garciaz (Cáceres) (Fig. 7.3). This memorial was conceived after a search for the human remains of 17 men and 2 women from the locality was unsuccessful. These men and women had presumably been killed and buried in the nearby village of Zorita, kilometres away from Garciaz, in 1936. One of the men in this group was the great-grandfather of historian Javier Martin Bastos, the researcher from PREMHEx in charge of the study of extrajudicial killings in the region (see Chap. 3). After several frustrated attempts to find the corpses, the families' association led by Javier decided to build a memorial in the cemetery of Garciaz using funds from the Ministry of the Presidency to carry out the reburial process. Javier did not consider the idea of building a memorial at the beginning—for the anger and distress he felt after the failed search made him want to forget the location and exhumation pursuit. With time, however, he and the other relatives agreed to place a commemorative headstone in Garciaz's cemetery.

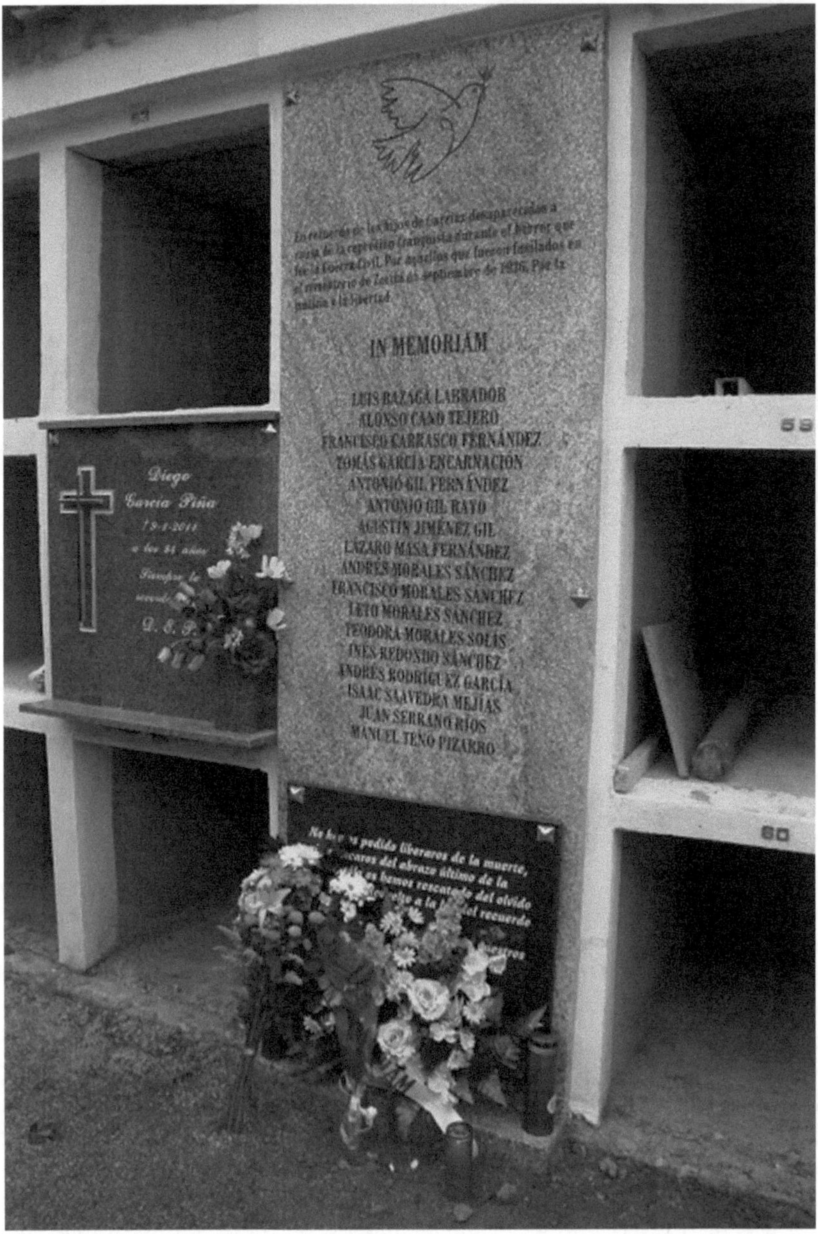

Fig. 7.3 Symbolic headstone on columbaria in the cemetery of Garciaz, in the province of Cáceres

For the association, and especially for Javier, who oversaw the memorial project, its construction was not a straightforward undertaking. Building the monument in the cemetery caused the researcher problems, not only with the village mayor and his Popular Party cabinet, but also with the Ministry that had awarded the funds to the families in the first place. On the one hand, the issue of the visibility and appearance of the tombstone became a point of contention again, as in Castuera case before the exhumation, between the association and Garciaz's conservative mayor. In contrast to the case of Puebla, when Javier tried to secure a plot in the cemetery, the mayor of Garciaz asked the families to buy three niches "in perpetuity," preferably located in a remote space of the burial ground. Hostile to the idea of having a commemorative site for the village's left-wing neighbours killed during the war, he advised Javier "not to write the cause of death" on the headstone "to avoid the discomfort of other village neighbours" and recommended that he opt for niches that were "less seeable" in the cemetery (Javier Martin Bastos, Cáceres 2012). Again, the inscription of their names and the epitaphs to their deaths awakened the anxiety of the local town hall, which understood the memorial as a subversive structure inside the cemetery. Even in the absence of bones and material belongings it was the abeyant social memory of the conflict that shaped the order of commemoration.

The construction of the structure led to further conflicts between the central government and the families' association. As Javier explained to me in an interview, after the project had been closed and half of the budget returned, due to the fruitless exhumation, the Ministry of the Presidency penalized the group, requesting an extra payment for spending funds dedicated to other activities in the original budget on the building of the memorial. The Ministry further supported their claim by stating "there was no need to build the memorial if the bodies had not been found" (Javier Martin Bastos, Cáceres 2012). Various conversations ensued between Javier and the state department, until the former decided to make a formal complaint regarding the government's decision, clarifying the budget imbalance and accompanying his statement with a report, which included, in his words, "historical, anthropological and psychological references to explain why the monolith should be built even if the human remains were not found" (ibid.). After this, Javier never heard back from the Ministry and took this administrative silence to be the end of the dispute. The process, Javier told me, exhausted him. Without knowledge of accounting or management of these administrative and legal procedures, he concluded that the arduous bureaucratic complications, together with the burdening tempo (Bourdieu 1979; Herzfeld 1991) of some administrative doings, first surrounding the exhumation project and later the building of the monolith, only exacerbated the fatigue and emotional weariness provoked by the inconclusive search for his relative's human remains. The body emerged as an ultimate form of material evidence needed in order to commemorate the past. Moreover, the state's requirements for a body to mourn evidenced the vagueness of the commitment to the memory of the conflict in national commemorative agendas.

The memorials in reburial processes, or commemorative events dedicated to the death of Republicans, gave place to a novelfunerary heritage in cemeteries with distinct spatial, aesthetic, and political signification (Young 1993). The presence of these buildings inside village graveyards reflected the collective endeavour of families and other groups to create a space for the mourning and remembrance of those killed as a result of Francoist repression. The intimate and enclosed public memory acts of these historical memory communities had distanced them from other modes and tropes of national tributes and celebrations. This novel burial heritage evokes different affiliations and is charged with the apprehensions and aspirations of families, activists, researchers, and state actors involved in their production. These memorial buildings are further signified in the context of the commemorative acts that envelop them. Here new idioms and rituals momentarily inhabit the cemetery, turning the space into a platform where familial bereavement, historical reclamation, and public denunciation converge.

The Rituals of Commemorative Reburials

The moment of the reburial of the corpses is often accompanied by a varied secular liturgy of acts in which families, association members, researchers, scientists and, at times, political representatives remember the deceased and their executions. Political and historical references interlace with the imagery created by the gestures, material manifestations, and messages enacted. In these acts, bodily practices—as Connerton (1989) termed them—and oral expressions entwine individual stories and experience with a wider concern for historical recognition and a demand for the state to *care* for the defeated and their families. They also, however, exposed the divergent desires of members of historical memory associations, who were not always unanimous in their thoughts about the reburial of the corpses. In the two acts that I attended in Garciaz in 2011 and Puebla de Alcocer in 2012, both ceremonies were marked by the results of the exhumation campaigns, the context in which the organization of the memorialisation project had taken place, and the visions that each individual had of the act of commemoration.

In Puebla de Alcocer, the act began with the movement of the corpses from the cemetery's autopsy room, where they had been briefly kept for the purpose of the tribute, to the mausoleum. In an emotive manner, relatives of the dead and some village neighbours carried the small wooden coffins that contained the corpses one by one, personally transporting them to their final resting place. Each box, decorated with a Republican flag and a red rose, was then placed next to the monolith while a cellist played classical pieces to accompany the event. Once the boxes were piled and arranged by the monument, some relatives, local politicians, and members of the research project read the texts they had prepared for the occasion. After the participants had spoken, a line of men and women, including the archaeologist, Laura Muñoz Encinar, passed the small boxes with the human remains to be deposited on the shelves inside the crypt of the mausoleum. The small number objects encountered in the mass graves were exhibited in the *Casa de la Cultura* (House of Culture), a village communal building, where personal belongings acquired the meaning of historical relics for the neighbours who went to visit them.

In Garciaz, the absence of the human remains of those buried in mass graves encouraged other ceremonial gestures and messages, from relatives and other participants in the project. The act brought together many neighbours from the town to uncover the granite gravestone listing the names of those who were killed. Members of the families' association stood next to the headstone, facing a crowd of people intensely engaging with this reencounter with the memory of defeat, at the symbolic reburial act on a cold day in December. Like in Puebla, relatives, mainly from third and fourth generations, recalled the stories of death that had been transmitted through their families over the years and read passages from books and the pieces they had written. Stories of repression were often interspersed with other references to the role of contemporary official institutions, reflecting the social tensions that surrounded the display of the headstone in Garciaz's cemetery. In both villages, reburial acts were followed by communal meals and other commemorative celebrations. In Puebla, those who organized the exhumation, together with the archaeologist Laura Muñoz Encinar, led an informative session in the village's *Casa de la Cultura* about the research and exhumation work carried out in the summer of 2012. In Garciaz, relatives read other passages and texts, in the intimacy of the restaurant salon that the families' association had hired for the gathering.

In both locations, these celebrations were civil ceremonies without religious symbols, homilies, or enactments, which instead drew on other material and discursive elements marked by the familial and political character of the burials. Nonetheless, in both cases issues around the type of ritual performed did emerge in connection to some relatives' particular desires for a more religious burial, as in the case of Puebla, or a more political ceremony, as in Garciaz. In both acts, however, subtle Republican imagery and political references were eventually preferred. As the town mayor of Puebla told me in our interview, the day was meant to be a day for the families and not one dominated by political speeches and messages from party representatives. In Puebla, flags were only used as attire for the coffins. Nevertheless, political messages were still heard, as not only relatives but also political agents took to the stage. In Garciaz, only some participants carried Republican symbols into the cemetery. As Javier had explained to me, however, some would have preferred a more visibly political ceremony. The character of the memorial and the event was thus a much-negotiated matter. Nevertheless, the messages that people transmitted generally addressed the Republican and left-wing identities of the dead and the political affiliations of the living, eliciting the importance of these left-wing histories in the contemporary political subjectivities of members from different generations and affiliations.

Just as the exhumation became a space of discreet commemoration, the realm of the funerary memorial emerged as an important place, where tributes to the dead were fervently performed. One could understand the significance of these rituals much in the way Durkheim once argued, for their capacity to integrate "individuals into communal life" (Metcalf and Huntington on Durkheim 1991, 28). Indeed the pressing demands for acknowledgement uttered by these collectives turned reburial events and their commemorative rites into bonding acts that sought the inclusion and continuity of a community of mourners for the war dead in the regulating social order. The tense relation between families, activists, and the state, however, exemplified how these events were more loci of resistance and disruption through which the strenuous ties with other groups and institutions could be devised. As Nadia Seremetakis (1991) suggests, drawing from the insights of historian Philippe Aries, death rites can be analysed as "deep structure" and regarded as a realm of "social contestation" (ibid., 14–15) in which distinct social entanglements can be explored. By taking the same approach, I propose, like her, to examine these performances around the war dead through the eyes, gestures, and words of the families and activists that take part in these reburial acts. In doing so, one can begin to understand the relevance these events gain for its participants not only as spaces to articulate a temporally dislocated commemoration of the war and postwar but also as a place where judicial, historical, and moral subjects are constituted in relation or opposition to the established social order. As Seremetakis contends, through this approach to ritual one can explore the institution of death as a "critical vantage point from which to view society" (ibid.).

In Garciaz and Puebla de Alcocer the messages expressed by those who publically addressed the crowd exemplified the important personal and social value many participants gave to these actions. In Puebla, for instance, the regional leader of PSOE at the time, Guillermo Fernandez Vara, who was invited by the town mayor and the families' association to attend the event, recognized that these acts provided the work of historical memory collectives with all its virtue and efficacy. As he implied, anyone who wants to understand what it means to talk about the historical memory of the war must attend a reburial event. For the PSOE leader it was coming into contact with families, when the human remains were returned to the cemetery, that the social significance of remembering the Civil War past could be gauged. In Garciaz, on the contrary, in the absence of human remains, Javier Martin Bastos ascertained that the importance of the event resided in the very act of returning their memory and, in particular, their names back to their village.

In both cases, these practices had a place-making capacity, for they consecrated a space for the deceased within the wider community of village dead (Connerton 1989). For many, these acts were the realization of a much longed-for yearning. As Consuelo Sánchez-Paniagua in Puebla de Alcocer noted, the reburial was the conclusion of years of waiting for José, her father, who finally lived to see the burial of his own father's human remains and the construction of the mausoleum. For others like Esperanza Muga Blasco's brother, Pedro, the act, which reunited him with his father, grandfather, and uncle's human remains, marked a beginning, rather than an end. For Paul Connerton (1989), the performance of ritual is embedded with a collective need to initiate new periods and social realities, to question the "trials of old regimes", and to constitute a new form of collective living. In the words of Pedro, reburial indeed marks a passage from a regime of occultation to one of disclosure through which the dead can have a respected place in the community of Puebla's dead. As he invoked during the event in Puebla:

> Today is a great day for us. It is a glorious Saturday because we have brought our ancestors where they needed to be, so everyone and all of us can know where and who are those who died for their democratic ideals in this village. Here, on this mausoleum, engraved with their names, a page about the Francoist disaster will be written for future generations. I want to remind you that today is not a day for mourning, for they already died and were already grieved... Today is a day for happiness because with this act, we accomplished their eternal rest next to other relatives and friends in this sacred place, where there are not ideological distinctions. It is a return to equality. (Pedro Muga Blasco, Puebla 2013)

As Pedro's words elucidate, the reburial ground is an important space for the making of a personal and collective history. Reburials allowed relatives to fix their history in time and space and express their own experiences of absence publically. In these ceremonies, personal feelings of bereavement often spoke of a common history of hardship with the deceased that marked familial trajectories. Many of these individual interventions were marked by intense emotion, expressed through the playfulness and poetics of the language used, which as Connerton (1989) has highlighted, is usually part of the performance and liturgy of commemorative rituals. In these contexts, such expressions sought to fulfil a personal tribute to the dead and also to strengthen the solemn character of these reburials in the public context in which they took place. These messages drew on the rhyme and weaving of their prose, on occasion addressing the dead directly to emphasize the proximity with them. For instance, when Pedro spoke to the gathered public, his words entangled his family's postwar fate with that of his father's, and summarized the profound connection he felt with his executed kin. As he expressed at the start of his speech:

> Hello father, you must like it when I call you father. The word sounds nice. I have never pronounced it in public. I do it today because I am again next to you, years after evil separated us, taking you away from home, to end with your life when I was four and my sister was two. However you and I know that, many times, crying about my mundane weaknesses I have called on you when I was alone. Just by saying 'Father!' you understood the content of my call. You have never stopped protecting me and with your help I overcame my problems. This is why some people said they have seen me alone but never crestfallen. They silenced your tongue with your death but not your sentiment that exists beyond life. I have always received your protection and with support and love of your wife, my mother, I have got through life uprightly in such a perverse situation… I send you a kiss and with all the love in the name of our family I receive your sacred human remains together with those of my grandfather and uncle, your father and brother. You will stay forever in this place, to rest eternally near your wife, who, like a heroine fulfilled her duties with your children, being a father and a mother, shaping my personality and smoothing any hatred over, to make me into a good citizen for society… (Pedro Muga Blasco, Puebla de Alcocer 2013)

The words Pedro dedicated to his father exemplified a need to proclaim and confess the impact of the relative's absence on the speaker's upbringing, on his life and personality. Faced by his father's human remains, he spoke to him as if they were meeting one last time before his reburial, to tell him he had never forgotten him. His warm recollection accentuated his dead father's affective presence in Pedro's day-to-day and in his reflective thoughts and introspection. His words made his families' suffering public, seeking to restore his father's virtue and legitimacy. Familial eulogies enacted a sense of duty and indebtedness with the dead. This kinship obligation also reflected many people's social and political commitment to honouring the causes for which their relatives lost their lives. As in Castuera, many of the texts and speeches pronounced in Puebla and Garciaz identified these men's deaths as the ultimate sacrifice for a democratic order—something that also resonated with forms and idioms of national and international war commemoration elsewhere (see Wagner 2013; Connerton 1989; Verdery 1999; Winter 1996; Anderson 1983).

Though Pedro expressed during his address that burying these men at the cemetery returned them to a "place where there [were] not ideological distinctions", these acts succinctly converted the location of the monolith into an arena where contemporary ideological beliefs were also conveyed, contested, and celebrated. Speakers' expressions often reflected individual experiences of the exhumation and memorialisation process and of the politics that surround these undertakings. In Puebla, for instance, many of the families who intervened thanked the town hall for its support in recovering the human remains and for enabling families' mourning. Though everyone agreed with the way the exhumation had been performed, many families also expressed concern with the way in which the human remains had been publically mourned. For instance, at the end of the act, in a crowded and stuffy room of the House of Culture, where people gathered to hear the presentation of results, Luisa Cabanillas Bayón stood up to ask why the ceremony at the cemetery had not been presided over by a priest. Luisa explained that she would have liked to have bid farewell to the human remains of her kin with a religious ceremony—just like the ceremonies other dead received before they were buried. The wishes of Luisa, of Catholic faith, indeed collided with those of other families and members of younger generations, for whom a civil ceremony seemed more suitable for burying the human remains of left-wing Republicans. At the event, the town mayor explained to Luisa that a non-religious burial had been chosen in accordance to the wish of the majority of the relatives that had been located. This incident revealed how the decision of a collective burial is often fraught with the conflicting visions of different participants and how the political traces of past identities and the political aspirations of present generations can shape the outcome of such commemorations.

In Garciaz, for instance, where relatives never found their kin's human remains, these messages were filled with an overreaching sense of pain and frustration for the inconclusive search and connected to disputes with local and national administrations around the building of the memorial. Here, written texts shared the space with spontaneous interactions from members of the public, who uttered their stories publically for the first time. During the event, Javier spoke of the long process the families had gone through in their search for the corpses. The archaeologist who led the location works, Sara Rodriguez Hidalgo, also addressed families, deeply afflicted by the impossibility of locating the mass grave. Many other people in the public intervened, identifying the names of the relatives, giving impromptu testimonies of their disappearance, and even cursing perpetrators—though names were never given. Many of the texts that had been prepared by relatives explicitly condemned past atrocities but also presented struggles, reclaiming the memory of their ancestors' deaths from the antagonistic political powers absent at the act. As Antonia Serrano Fernandez, the granddaughter of one of the men who disappeared, expressed in the text she composed for the event:

> No one should see this act as a revanchist endeavour or simply to stir up the past. Some people talk about opening old wounds, but in what heart is that wound? Is it in the executioner's or in victims and families' hearts? They should only see it as an act of justice. It's about building a future for all but not over an interested forgetting or over an imposed collective amnesia. We have tried to get them out of the place where they threw them in the most ignominious way but so far, the excavations carried out have been fruitless and certainly, our possibilities are each time more remote… Today, the remains of our loved ones are not behind these nameplates, there is only the metaphorical emptiness of their absence… This [monument] will remain as space for memory and against the atrocities provoked by war, especially wars that confront brothers against brothers and neighbours against neighbours. We are going to have the honour to remember them with this act and to leave proof that they were murdered with impunity, without an accusation or the possibility of a just defence. They were killed in 'Luca's Sewer', in the farm called 'el Zorro', between Zorita and Logrosán, on the road to Conquista, in Cáceres, in the "Roble" and in other yet undefined places… They all died defending their ideas of social progress embedded in the Second Republic, with its virtues and flaws. But especially they died defending democracy and freedom; we honour their memory today… (Antonia Serrano Fernandez, Garciaz 2011)

At the commemorative act, stories of repression acquired, to recall Julie Cruikshank's (1998) expression, other social lives as part of the rights petitions and endeavours of civil society collectives. Their retelling at the event was a way of providing evidence about the reality of the killings, the suffering of the families, and the need for remembrance—even if the bodies had not been found. In this setting, as Paul Connerton (1989, 58) has observed, liturgy, with its imperative force, was a potent call to action and a response to the expressions of the official institution—back then under the government of PSOE—and the local PP representative: a proposition to actively engage with this history publically for participants at the event and, most importantly, for those beyond the realm of the commemorative space. Ritual choices also revealed that the controversies of these acts were imbued with both intimate and public interests in signifying the human remains of the Republican dead. The civil ritual chosen by relatives, however, shared many commonalities with other commemorative ceremonies elsewhere—see for instance the still prominent D-Day and World War I celebrations, or the Holocaust Memorial Day ceremonies around the world. The use of certain material forms, bodily performances, and literary and oratory styles evoked their historicity and their relation to similar historical memory events in other parts of the country.

The commemorative reburials I attended in Extremadura stood out for the innovative practices, designs, and idioms they incorporated to remember the deaths of left-wing Republicans. The form and meanings of their monuments and acts were intricately ensnared with the social context in which they took place, on the margins of national memorialisation, and in connection with varied desires for historical validation. Their secular character provided them with a different quality in the realm of the cemetery, reflecting the role that these commemorative occasions played as important scenarios where civil, political, and moral demands were enacted. Certainly, some families I met still preferred a combined funeral officiated by a priest to worship the dead in the Catholic tradition. For many others, the civil acts that accompanied the funerary monuments and re-interments represented the wishes of most participants, who preferred a non-confessional ceremony—as for many, the values of the Second Republic did not tally with the doctrines and involvement of the Catholic Church in the conflict and ensuing dictatorship. Nonetheless, collective reburials and commemoration sought to return the human remains of the Republican killed to the cemetery to make their memory sacred. These acts and the material inscriptions in the cemetery gained significance as performative and symbolic manifestations of the recollection of such a traumatic past in the present. For many, they will remain documents—part of a growing surrogate archive—that testify to the horrors of the Civil War and the social experience of different generations. Reburial acts became another space where historical knowledge about the executions was assembled, and where a new culture of bereavement was articulated by the heterogeneous community of mourners that came together in concern for left-wing supporters executed during and after the Civil War.

Note

1. In Extremadura mortal remains are returned to families or the associations that promote the exhumation and reburial. As an activity regulated by the Law of Patrimony in the region, however, the outcomes of these exhumations are also overseen by the administration. As opposed to what is advised in the national protocol, bodies in the region are usually buried without their belongings. Following article 53 (e) of the Law of

Patrimony, and as a measure to secure their protection, objects are be kept at the pertinent provincial museum in the absence of direct relatives to recover them.

References

Anderson, Benedict R. 1983. *Imagined Communities: Reflections on the Origin and Spread of Nationalism*. London: Verso.

Bourdieu, Pierre. 1979. *Outline of a Theory of Practice*. Cambridge: Cambridge University Press.

Buckham, Susan. 2003. Commemoration as an Expression of Personal Relationship and Group Identities: A Case Study of York Cemetery. *Mortality* 8 (2): 160–175.

Connerton, Paul. 1989. *How Societies Remember*. Cambridge: Cambridge University Press.

Cruikshank, Julie. 1998. *The Social Life of Stories: Narrative and Knowledge in the Yukon Territory*. Lincoln: University of Nebraska Press.

Exteberría, Francisco et al. 2012. Exhumación, identificación y causa de muerte en la fosa común de Aibar-Oibar (Navarra). *Munibe (Antropología-Arkeología)* 63: 367–377.

Foltyn, Jacque Lynn. 2008. Dead Famous and Dead Sexy: Popular Culture, Forensics, and the Rise of the Corpse. *Mortality* 13 (2): 153–173.

Gell, Alfred. 1999. The Technology of Enchantment and Enchantment of Technology. In *The Art of Anthropology: Essays and Diagrams*, ed. Eric Hirsch, 159–186. Cambridge: Cambridge University Press.

Granjel, Mercedes, and Antonio Carreras Panchón. 2004. Extremadura y el debate sobre la creación de cementerios: un problema de salud pública en la ilustración. *Norba. Revista de Historia* 17: 69–91.

Herzfeld, Michael. 1991. *A Place in History: Social and Monumental Time in a Cretan Town*. Princeton, NJ: Princeton University Press.

Jelin, Elizabeth, and Victoria Langland. 2003. *Monumentos, memoriales y marcas territoriales*. Madrid: Siglo Veintiuno de España Editores; Buenos Aires: Siglo Veintiuno de Argentina Editores.

Kwon, Heonik. 2006. *After the Massacre: Commemoration and Consolation in Ha My and My Lai*. Berkeley, CA: University of California Press.

Kwon, Heonik. 2008. *Ghosts of War in Vietnam*. Cambridge: Cambridge University Press.

Laqueur, Thomas W. 1994. Memory and Naming in the Great War. In *Commemorations: The Politics of National Identity*, ed. John R. Gillis. Chichester: Princeton University Press.

Metcalf, Peter, and Richard Huntington. 1991. *Celebrations of Death: The Anthropology of Mortuary Ritual*. Cambridge: Cambridge University Press.

Petrović-Šteger, Maja. 2012. Mobile Sepulchre and Interactive Formats of Memorialization: On Funeral and Mourning Practices in Digital Art. *Journeys* 13 (2): 71–89.

Presidency, Ministry of the. 2011. Orden PRE/2568/2011, de 26 de septiembre, por la que se publica el Acuerdo del Consejo de Ministros de 23 de septiembre de 2011, por el que se ordena la publicación en el Boletín Oficial del Estado del Protocolo de actuación en exhumaciones de víctimas de la guerra civil y la dictadura. *Boletín Oficial del Estado.*

Rios, Luis, Juan Ignacio Casado and Jorge Puente Prieto. 2010. Identification Process in the Mass Graves from the Spanish Civil War. *Forensic Science International*, 199 (1–3): E27–E36.

Rugg, Julie. 2003. Introduction: Cemeteries. *Mortality* 8 (2): 107–112.

Seremetakis, Nadia C. 1991. *The Last Word: Women, Death, and Divination in Inner Mani.* Chicago: University of Chicago Press.

Verdery, Katherine. 1999. *The Political Lives of Dead Bodies: Reburial and Postsocialist Change.* New York: Columbia University Press.

Wagner, Sarah E. 2008. *To Know Where He Lies: DNA Technology and the Search for Srebrenica's Missing.* Berkeley, CA and London: University of California Press.

Wagner, Sarah E. 2013. The Making and Unmaking of an Unknown Soldier. *Social Studies of Science* 43 (5): 631–656.

Wagner, Sarah E. 2014. The Social Complexities of Commingled Remains. In *Commingled Human Remains: Methods in Recovery, Analysis and Identification*, ed. B. Adams and J. Byrd. New York: Academic Press.

Winter, Jay M. 1996. *Sites of Memory, Sites of Mourning: the Great War in European Cultural History.* Cambridge: Cambridge University Press.

Young, James E. 1993. *The Texture Of Memory: Holocaust Memorials and Meaning.* New Haven: Yale University Press.

CHAPTER 8

The Exhumation as Emerging Archive

Exhumation processes have opened up new avenues for research into the history of the Spanish Civil War—not only in Extremadura but also in the rest of the country. The task of searching for information about the Republican executed and missing, excavating their human remains, and reburying their corpses in cemeteries has triggered the emergence of new epistemologies around the traces of the violence of Francoist repression. In this process, the meanings of past historical regimes have been confronted and also redefined, in an endeavour to reclaim the names, histories, and bodies of those who lost the war. When I went to Extremadura to study exhumations, I observed how scientific practice, familial recollection, and archival research convened to produce new types of enunciation, in order to challenge past official narratives and political realities. Such processes revealed other relations and information networks that were in the making, through which the identity of the missing was negotiated and constructed, socially. To me, the activities in which families, archaeologists, historians, and activists engaged in order to produce knowledge about the war past seemed to delineate the contours of a new archive, which, as Michel Foucault (1972, 130) observes, constitutes an alternative "general system" in which new statements are formed and transformed. As seen throughout this book, thinking and tracing this new archive sheds light on the way in which these exhumations aimed to re-signify the violent and obscured deaths of the Republican defeated in the war. It also, however, elucidated new

Z. Aragüete-Toribio, *Producing History in Spanish Civil War Exhumations*, World Histories of Crime, Culture and Violence,
DOI 10.1007/978-3-319-61270-6_8

political subjectivities that were still in the making and the emergence of different political spaces where those affected by such history of loss articulated their claims and concerns.

In order to understand the reach and importance of the act of unearthing these human remains in the present, we have to return to the moment when violence erupted, and to the aftermath of the war. The exhumations of the twenty first century in Spain, as we have seen, cannot be taken in isolation as bounded events but must instead be considered in relation to the treatment that the Republican body—whether dead or alive—received over time. The scientific, legal, mnemonic, and political regimes that formed around these human remains in the past decade speak directly of the sovereignty of past governments, of their memory politics, and of the social imagination that has existed around the war victory and defeat. The event of the exhumation can be traced back to the decades before the conflict, to clashes of different mentalities and moralities at a time of extreme social inequality. Locating the history of the Republican body hence elucidates past differences, which are often connected to present struggles around the so-called "recovery" of the memory of the conflict.

Chapter 2 showed how dominant ideologies shaped the political pulse of the country, pacts made during the transition to democracy, and the culture of consensus that has prevailed in the country since 1975 have been challenged in social, political judicial and historical realms. Unearthing the human remains of the Republican executed in 2000 led to the contestation of hegemonic positions surrounding the memory of the conflict, demanding political and social transformation. Certainly at a national level, as seen in the cases of ARMH and the Foro, and in the case of other regional collectives in Extremadura, the associations that promote these exhumations in the present have opened a new civil space and created a new voice, which draws on the language of international human rights and on the example of other countries, where transitional justice models have been applied. In their appeals, there is a desire to destabilize old amnesty agreements and pacts of silence, to press for recognition of the Republican victims, and to acknowledge their story in the collective history of the country. Campaigns such as those taken to the UN and others that, at a national level, condemned the oppressive law of the dictatorial regime and its abuses, undermined the transitional status quo and demanded the active involvement of the Spanish judicial and administrative institutions. Over the years, these associations have battled to dismantle old regimes of truth, altering and influencing past and present state decisions, regional regulations, and local politics.

The search into official and personal archives, the gathering of testimonies, and the archaeological and anthropological study of mass graves has allowed for other forms knowledge production, and situated historical research and writing at the centre of this social project. Some of these actions only became possible through the visibility the movement acquired in the last decade. The declassification of state documents, the appearance of new witness' accounts, and the opening of mass graves have all been affected by the contexts in which they have occurred. The level of involvement of different governments throughout the years, with the passing of the so-called Law of Historical Memory in 2007 under the PSOE government and the dismantling of all measures since the election of the right-wing PP in 2011, has most certainly shaped the conditions and experience of assembling an alternative narrative of the Republican past. Limited aid from the central administration at different moments has meant a lack of a centralized and consistent approach to these searches. Leaving the work of investigation and exhumation to independent actors, associations and, on occasions, particular institutions, led to the formation of very heterogeneous approaches to such process of inquiry. In comparison to post-conflict scenarios elsewhere, the Spanish case reveals how these independent exhumation and memorialisation strategies, crafted as part of a bottom–up approach (Ferrándiz 2013) to reparation, are constantly negotiated between the desires of individuals and local, regional, and national associations and institutions.

As discussed in Chap. 3, early on in my fieldwork, I realized that different political, scientific, and social realities and aspirations affected the production of history and such novel processes of information gathering. In Extremadura, the political agreement between different institutions since 2003, first under the PSOE government and then after 2011, to a lesser extent, under the regional administration of the Popular Party, secured the ongoing research carried out by historians and archaeologists from PREMHEx, part of the University of Extremadura. Such a platform, which did not exist in every region, facilitated the work of compilation and research into forms of Francoist repression, but also the location, exhumation, identification, and reburial of human remains. Nonetheless, after the Popular Party took over the regional government, many of these projects were delayed and postponed. Different institutional backing provided particular frameworks for the historical memory enterprise in the region. For over a decade, institutional aid mostly facilitated a space in which the information gathered from archives, but also testimonies and exhumations, could be centralized, analysed, digitized, and made available publically. It also prompted regulation of exhumations by the Heritage Law, providing a way of legally and officially accounting for these actions. These initiatives, however, were sometimes at odds with the wishes of historical memory associations and families in the area. As seen in Chaps. 4 and 5, on occasions, the project's work was contested by the wishes of local associations, and the bureaucratic demands and time exigencies of a Heritage Law that often clashed with the urgency of exhumation projects and the needs of archaeological teams and historical memory groups.

These exhumation projects aimed to establish a new type of research and modus operandi that addressed the lack of informed institutional backing, devising protocols and guidelines in the absence of a national historical memory plan. They also aimed to formalise the character of historical inquiry into the war past realized in the region. As seen in Chap. 3, the specific approach that PREMHEx took to the investigation of the conflict placed strong emphasis on the production of objective knowledge. This was partly connected to the professional profiles of researchers, widely trained in the fields of history and archaeology and in their particular methodologies. It was also connected to a desire of producing a type of knowledge detached from specific ideological dictums or subjective involvement. Nonetheless, the treatment of the archive, of testimonies, and of mass graves, was also, as members of the project agreed, intertwined with a humanitarian desire to help families and support associations and as such, with a strong personal will to implement and help to realize historical memory demands (as Renshaw 2011 has also pointed out). In such a way, the work of scientists was entangled with personal motivations often linked to private histories and a social commitment to elucidate what happened during and after the war. Objectivity and methodological precision were tools for the acquisition of a kind of truth—a truth that enlightened the effects of Francoist violence in order to legitimate war and postwar histories of suffering on the part of Republican relatives and survivors, as well as to accredit the project's work, the quality of the research produced, and the authenticity of these results in a landscape where multiple visions of the past coexisted.

The ethnographic cases presented in Chaps. 4 and 5 exemplify how the exhumation site was a space in which interaction between different methods, knowledge, and intentions occurred, where different actors converged, and diverse versions of history proliferated. For the historians and archaeologists at PREMHEx, these two sites were part of a broader map of excavations, through which repression patterns in the region could be discerned. The unearthing of these human remains was also entangled with the relations between PSOE, IU, and PP in the region, and long searches on the part of local families. The comparison I have drawn between these two exhumation projects showed how the traces of the missing in documents, stories, and inside the mass grave gained different meanings. Both cases demonstrated how temporal distance and uncertainty, which underlies the whole process of searching for the dead and their histories, was negotiated for particular purposes. Traces were examined and spoken about in order to generate certainty about the executions and compose lasting narratives from scientific evidence, analysis of the archive, the story of witnesses, and inherited accounts of second, third, and fourth generations of relatives and neighbours. In each context, however, the presence or absence of material and bodily remains, the existence of relatives connected to the corpses, or the memories of the killings shaped the experience of death and disappearance.

In Castuera, the appearance of numerous human remains, unknown to researchers, family relatives, or the archive, prompted an inquiry within which archaeological and physical anthropology analyses guided the interpretation of the mass grave, defining the identities of the human remains and their relation to the concentration Camp that once existed outside the village. The bones—and in particular the objects found—were viewed in correlation with the testimonies that the historian had previously gathered from ex-prisoners and witnesses, and with documents from official registries and archives, in order to "fill in the blanks" of the historical record. Scientific information helped to establish a narrative about the Camp, reasserting its existence and turning the materiality of the mass grave into evidence of the events and killings that occurred during the postwar period. It also attributed to these corpses a possible identity, defining their human persona—for instance, through the objects they carried. For researchers, this meant a development in the creation of a history of the Camp. For historical memory activists, who supported the exhumation, acquiring such scientific evidence was a way of claiming entitlement over the re-writing of the village's past in a contested local political arena. For the families of those who were detained and were never found, the human remains and objects in the mass grave evoked stories of long-gone relatives and the impossibility of their return. In the interplay between bones, storytelling, and scientific interpretation, archaeological constructions of the mass grave led young activists to reclaim the political identities of these human remains, and prompted families to reconsider the fate of their relatives.

The presence and materiality of corpses and their adjacent objects, once exposed in the excavation process, unleashed a plethora of first-hand and transmitted memories, which in turn unveiled the kinship and social relations of the dead and the powerful social life of these stories of repression in the present. In the case of Puebla de Alcocer, discussed in Chap. 5, stories transmitted about the killings throughout generations were an important element in the scientific analysis of the mass grave. Stories negotiated the meanings lent to the space by scientific practices and the archive, and the force of the mass graves became apparent as people tried to relate new scientific information to the version of the execution story they had always known. The limited information found in the mass grave, due to the badly-preserved bodily and material remains, meant that storytelling became a way of situating and contextualizing the killings for the scientists. Political alliances or conflict between neighbours before the war mixed with stories of repression that recalled the way in which people had been killed. Stories depicted the traits of individuals in the mass grave, identifying their familial, social, and political personas and pointing to the link that present generations felt with the deceased. These accounts had a capacity to instil a sense of time and continuity for some relatives, but also contrasted with the silence of others, who felt reticent about speaking by the graveside. They also provided families with a sense of historicity within the community, and revealed how individuals imagined themselves in time and as part of the village's collective life. Stories, as Cruickshank (1998) has argued, reunited younger and older generations over the sharing of the past.

The mass graves in Puebla and Castuera became spaces of transmission between generations, in which emerging stories—but also new scientific interpretations—were incorporated into the memory of the event. Exchanges between neighbours, scientists, and relatives led to the reassertion of local interpretations of the executions, but also turned other visions into mythical constructions. Scientific analysis, but also the sight of the skeletons and their dispositions, challenged the assumptions and veracity of some accounts—for instance,

and in particular, those of survival, which were marked by the ambivalence that a disappearance triggers (Domanska 2005). The making and unmaking of the event by relatives, activists, scientists, volunteers, and visitors turned the space of interaction between experts and non-experts. The mass grave became a space in which the interaction between bones, documents and objects, and the living erased the distinction between science and politics, between the knowledge of archaeologists, historians, activists and families, and between people and things. At the mass grave, moreover, a political ontology emerged—in Latour's sense—around new matters of concern, which diverged from the political culture fostered since the transition to democracy and was affected by the heavy weight that the past had placed on the lives of different generations.

The force of the postmemory of these events motivated the impulse through which the past was continually re-invented by the graveside. The emergence of these new objects triggered a need to know and to grasp a past that could not be fully comprehended. This drive to make history was, in my view, fuelled by a war past that could be felt even if it had not been lived, and which expanded through time to become part of the everyday lives of the living during the postwar period and the time of the exhumation. The presence of these uncovered traces of violence evoked an image of the disappeared and executed, a reminder of their absence and a will to apprehend their experience. Images, documents, bones and objects were indexical of the person that was killed, though only in fragmented and partial ways. These offered hazy glimpses of fatal encounters with death and an unfinished vision of their fate. The encounters with the materiality of the archive and that of the grave generated other expressions of the uncanny, exposing the uncertain histories of past relatives, militants and members of the community in different contexts. Families, scientists and others were moved by the urge to solve what these images and objects "lacked"—recalling W.J.T. Mitchell (1996)—what they could not show and that the living desired to know. They were, as I explored in Chap. 6, moved by the affective force of violence, which permeated the actions, feelings, and emotions of people for years and conditioned the most intimate searches for clues about the killings in the present.

These forms of making history are not ordinary endeavours but efforts enmeshed with an unresolved experience of trauma, caused by the absence of bodies, the absence of signs, and an elusive historical imagination. To speak about the crafting of history in relation to the exhumation of the Republican killed, I argued—like Veena Das (2007)—is to consider how particular forms of violence have affected individuals and collectivities over time. It also means considering how such violence, which emanated from the desecrated corpses of the defeated, has haunted political measures and decisions, neighbourly interactions, and personal subjective worlds—from the moment in which it was perpetrated until today. Biographical accounts revealed parts of a history that had rarely been spoken about. They also, however, exposed the ways in which past hardship had been internalized and performed, thus continuing to affect subsequent generations. The traces that remained of these killings made history thinkable both for the historian and the relative. Documents and images, bones and objects were charged with an aura of repression, a trail of fear, and visible signs of reppresive postwar politics. When considering these alternative modes of enunciation (Rancière 1994), one ought to think of how the latent anguish trapped in these vestiges shaped the experiences of those who engaged with them. On the one hand, one should consider how their affective force led people to embark on incessant and prolonged searches for their ancestors in official and personal archives and mass graves, in order to reconstruct an image and memory that challenged their absence. On the other hand, one should also try to appreciate how these traces, which contain fraudulent representations and violent inscriptions, unsettles the person that searches, making the endeavour for history an distressing yet consoling affair.

The production of the history and the recovery of the corpses of the Republican dead are also imbued with strong moral sentiments and a desire to honour their memory and rebury their corpses. At the exhumation ground, the treatment of the human remains was directly entwined with the personal and political wishes of families, activists, and the exhumation team. Their recovery was ultimately connected to a desire to return these bodies to the safe space of the community and to see their reburial in the cemetery. Scientific technologies have acquired a central role as modes of accounting, collecting, and identifying human remains in Spain. Many families and activists have regarded the scientific excavation of the mass graves as an intricate and laborious process and admired the time and dedication of the teams with which I worked during my fieldwork. Techniques, such as DNA analysis, have proved, as Wagner (2008) has observed, to be a "technology of repair", which has reunited different generations and re-established kinship bonds through biological reconstructions. The rituals followed during reburials, the transportation of coffins, the attire of boxes, the mausoleums and tombstones built, and the speeches performed during these occasions, have created a new culture around the corpses and the memory of the Republican executed and estranged at the periphery of state action. Like exhumations, reburials also constituted a space in which familial and political wishes were pursued through the aid of scientific scrutiny.

As discussed in Chap. 7, reburials reunited a community around the defeated, with a common interest in commemorating their lives and contesting past and present national political agendas. These communities shared a common vision—though in practice, they often entertained heterogeneous goals and desires. Reburials—just like exhumation processes—often reflected how different political and familial wishes diverged in relation to the mortuary rites. As seen in the case of Castuera, Puebla, and Garciaz—where some families preferred individual to collective burials, political symbols, or religious over civil ceremonies—the decisions made by these groups were taken collectively and often influenced by the wishes of a majority, though the process was often fraught also with disagreements. Reburials provided a space in which collective memory and imagination could be performed, but also, in which conflict between historical memory actors manifested. The building of memorials and the re-interment also created a forum of denunciation, where the frictions between these civil-society collectives and governmental entities at local, regional, and national level were made apparent and contested. The staging of these memorials elicited, as shown in the last chapter, the motivations and desires of a community in localized areas and at particular moments in time. Authors like Young (1993) have shown, however, that memorials can lose their meaning with the passing of time, and can come to be re-signified by future generations. Whereas some of the memorials built around Extremadura in the last decade symbolize this particular moment, not all of them have continued to be used for collective commemoration. Many have remained tokens of private mourning and individual remembrance.

The exhumation and reburial of these human remains is still today, at the time of writing, driven by the ethical concerns of historical memory associations, families, volunteers, and independent scientific teams, which have generated an established exhumation practice over nearly two decades. The beginning of the Popular Party government in 2011, however, made the continuation of exhumations and historical memory campaigns extremely difficult and their existence became more precarious. While at the start of its mandate the party agreed that funds would still be available for the historical memory project, later discourses of austerity and a general lack of interest on the part of the new government ended all financial aid for exhumations and the cessation of grants for identification and reburials. In this context, today, many of the national historical memory associations—such as ARMH or the Foro—have resorted to independent fundraising tactics, using crowdfunding to fund searches and excavations that relatives still widely demand. Limited funds have led to a decrease in the number of exhumations, which are now funded by private and, on some occasions, international donors. The progressive absence of support on the part of national and regional bodies has also led to the threat of closure of laboratories, and has called into question the permanence of projects and associations around the country. Moreover, the passivity of the central government has only strengthened the reticent positions of judges and institutions, which have continued to reject and deter recent petitions for the accountability and trial of Francoist perpetrators.

Recent developments demonstrate the influence that political and legal decisions have in the process of exhumation, reburial, and commemoration of human remains. They also show how the past remains an asset in current political scenarios. In Extremadura, for instance, the relation of PP and IU at a regional level—which was forged after the regional election of 2011—triggered new changes in PREMHEx and transformed its team by the end of 2014. The new Project for the Recovery of Historical Memory in Extremadura would have a different lead investigator and exhumations' coordinator. Some mentioned that these actions were prompted by the desire of particular individuals to open up the research of the past to other historians outside of the university. Others explained that there were personal interests that clashed in relation to how the research into the Civil War past and the exhumation of mass graves should be conducted. Some activists to whom I spoke at the time were concerned about the fact that, with this arrangement, PP managed to reduce the impact of the project, as well as its activity. Many believed that behind these actions there was a desire on the part of the right-wing party to eventually dismantle any regional institutional support for the investigation into the conflict.

Political decisions had also a direct impact on the writing of some of the results of the previous project. Though Javier and Candela, the two PhD historians who worked for PREMHEx, submitted their theses before the end of the project, Laura's work was not finalised at that point. Hired as an archaeologist and never as a PhD researcher for the project, the researcher struggled to complete the analysis of some corpses, the writing of final reports, and the final writing of her thesis without full institutional backing. The new project had also been clear about the change of direction the new investigation would take. This new direction opened up a process of inquiry, with new aims, methods, and objectives, which decentralized the work of the university and involved other research actors. This would constitute a new form of investigation in the region, which would most certainly trigger the articulation of other discursive formations and practices around the war past in connection to the emergent exhumation archive. For many, the lack of funds for exhumations has led, in the last years, to an inability to attend, support, and accomplish pending demands for reparation made by many families.

The future of historical memory initiatives and exhumations seems uncertain today in Extremadura but also in the rest of Spain. Understanding the production of the history of the civil conflict in the present is crucial in order to discern how the past manifests in the social, political, and familial worlds of contemporary subjects. I have aimed to show that writing the history of the war means contesting old regimes of truth—but also present political discourses and practices. Exhumation processes have certainly triggered new ways of relating to the war, which have brought together activists, politicians, scientists, and families. They have triggered the emergence of artefacts and stories, charged with meanings and feelings of past suffering, which have in turn prompted the formation of alternative spaces for knowledge production and enabled new avenues of political action. In the light of the most recent developments in the region and around the country, one can begin to appreciate the temporal dynamics of such systems of historical enunciation: a new archive that was set in motion continues to be altered through the conflicting desires among the living and the presence of the dead. The production of history—its inner workings and outer manifestations—has become significant in order to understand both how individuals and collectivities negotiate their past in this emerging milieu, through the creation of idioms, spaces and practices that reconfigure their common and private lives.

References

Cruickshank, Julie. 1998. *The Social Life of Stories: Narrative and Knowledge in the Yukon Territory*. Vancouver: University of British Columbia Press.

Das, Veena. 2007. *Life and Words: Violence and the Descent into the Ordinary*. Berkeley: University of California Press.

Domanska, Ewa. 2005. Toward the Archaeontology of the Dead Body. In *Rethinking History* 9: 389–413.

Ferrándiz, Francisco. 2013. Exhuming the Defeated: Civil War Mass Graves in 21st Century Spain. *American Ethnologist* 40 (1): 38–54.

Foucault, Michel, and Alan Sheridan. 1972. *The Archaeology of Knowledge*. London: Tavistock Publications.

Latour, Bruno. 1999. *Pandora's Hope: Essays on the Reality of Science Studies*. London: Harvard University Press.

Mitchell, W. J . T. 1996. What Do Pictures 'Really' Want?, *October* 77: 71–82.

Rancière, Jacques. 1994. *The Names of History: On the Poetics of Knowledge*. Minneapolis: University of Minnesota Press.

Renshaw, Layla. 2011. *Exhuming Loss: Memory, Materiality and Mass Graves of the Spanish Civil War*. Calif: Left Coast.

Wagner, Sarah E. 2008. *To Know Where He Lies: DNA Technology and the Search for Srebrenica's Missing*. Berkeley, CA and London: University of California Press.

Young, James E. 1993. *The Texture of Memory: Holocaust Memorials and Meaning*. New Haven and London: Yale University Press.

Index

Z. Aragüete-Toribio, *Producing History in Spanish Civil War Exhumations*, World Histories of Crime, Culture and Violence,
DOI 10.1007/978-3-319-61270-6

FSC
www.fsc.org
MIX
Papier | Fördert gute Waldnutzung
FSC® C083411

Kolibri 360 GmbH
Ferdinand-Jühlke-Straße 7
99095 Erfurt, Deutschland
produktsicherheit@kolibri360.de